MW01517987

TOTAL FITNESS
EXERCISE, NUTRITION, AND WELLNESS

SCOTT K. POWERS
STEPHEN L. DODD
THE UNIVERSITY OF FLORIDA

ALLYN AND BACON
BOSTON · LONDON · TORONTO · SYDNEY · TOKYO · SINGAPORE

ISBN 0-205-18310-7

Printed in the United States of America

10 9 8 7 6 5 4 3 2 1   00 99 98 97 96

Preface

This instructor's manual is designed to assist the instructor of physical fitness and wellness in preparation of lecture materials, exams, and laboratory experiences. This manual contains a chapter summary, learning objectives, and a lecture outline for each chapter of *Total Fitness: Exercise, Nutrition, and Wellness* . In addition, a list of suggested class and laboratory experiences is included as well as a test bank.

The lecture outline follows the sequence of topics presented in the text. This outline provides a list of key points, and each key point is expanded by a list of subpoints. Many of the subpoints are illustrated via examples or additional details that might be useful to the beginning student of fitness and wellness. The outline is followed by a list of suggested laboratory experiences which assists the instructor in illustrating specific concepts in physical fitness and wellness. These lab experiences are designed to provide the instructor with ideas for practical laboratory experiences to aid the student in self evaluation and/or learning specific concepts in fitness and wellness. Next, discussion activities, suggested student activities, and supplemental readings are provided to help the instructor in planning class activities. Finally, a test bank of over 700 questions is provided which contains multiple choice, true/false, and discussion questions that are intended for use with the undergraduate student. Correct answers, a page reference, and type of question (factual or conceptual) follow each question.

TABLE OF CONTENTS

Chapter 5 - Improving Muscular Strength and Endurance

Chapter 6 - Improving Flexibility

Chapter 7 - Nutrition, Health, and Fitness

Chapter 15 - Sexually Transmitted Diseases and Drug Abuse

Chapter 16 - Lifetime Fitness

Chapter 1

Understanding Health-Related Physical Fitness and Wellness

CHAPTER SUMMARY

1. Exercise offers many health benefits. Regular exercise has been shown to reduce risk of CHD and diabetes, increase bone mass, and maintain physical working capacity during normal aging.

2. The five major components of "total" health-related physical fitness are:
   1) cardiorespiratory endurance
   2) muscular strength
   3) muscular endurance
   4) flexibility
   5) body composition

3. The term wellness means "healthy living". This state of healthy living is achieved by the practice of a positive health life style which includes regular physical activity, proper nutrition, eliminating unhealthy behaviors (avoiding high risk activities such as reckless driving, smoking, and drug use), and maintaining good emotional and spiritual health.

4. Total wellness can only be achieved by a balance of physical, emotional, intellectual, spiritual, and social health. The components of wellness do not work in isolation; there is a strong interaction among the five. For example, poor physical health can lead to poor emotional health. Similarly, a lack of spiritual health can contribute to poor emotional health, as well as poor physical health.

5. Exercise goal-setting is a key component in the maintenance of a lifetime fitness program.

LEARNING OBJECTIVES

After studying this chapter, you should be able to:

1. Describe the health benefits of exercise.
2. Define the terms "coronary artery disease" and "myocardial infarction".
3. Compare the goals of health-related fitness programs and sport performance conditioning programs.
4. Describe the components of health-related physical fitness.
5. Discuss the wellness concept.
6. Outline the components of wellness.

LECTURE OUTLINE

Key Points	Subpoints	Examples
Health benefits of exercise	1. Reduced risk of heart disease	
	2. Reduced risk of diabetes	Lower incidence of type II diabetes
	3. Exercise increases bone mass	
	4. Maintenance of work capacity	Improved quality of life
	5. Exercise increases longevity	
Exercise does not guarantee good health	1. Physically fit people can develop disease	Many factors (i.e. age, environment, genetics, life style, etc.) contribute to the risk of disease
Components of health-related physical fitness	1. cardiorespiratory fitness	Ability to perform vigorous exercise
	2. muscular strength	Lifting a maximal weight
	3. muscular endurance	Performing multiple repetitions
	4. flexibility	Joint mobility
	5. body composition	% body fat
Wellness concept	state of healthy living	Maximizing emotional, social, intellectual, and spiritual health and reducing the risk of disease and accidents

Key Points	Subpoints	Examples
Components of wellness	1. Physical health	Physical fitness and freedom from disease
	2. Emotional health	Emotional stability
	3. Intellectual health	Keeping an active mind
	4. Spiritual health	Ability to experience love, joy, peace, and to care and respect all living things
	5. Social health	Maintaining meaningful interpersonal relationships
Exercise goal setting	1. Goal setting is important in maintaining a life-long commitment to exercise	Goal setting maintains motivation
Key points in goal setting	1. Establish achievable goals	
	2. Put goals in writing	
	3. Establish both short-term and long-term goals	
	4. Goals should be measurable	
	5. Set target dates for achievement of goals	
	6. After goal achievement, establish another goal	
	7. Reward yourself after achievement of a goal	

LAB ACTIVITIES

LABORATORY 1.1 (pages 15-16)

Students should complete *Lifestyle assessment inventory* laboratory (Laboratory 1-1). The purpose of this laboratory is to increase individual awareness of areas in lifestyle that increase the risk of accidents and disease.

DISCUSSION ACTIVITIES

• Organize small student discussion groups to critically evaluate the individual components that comprise the concept of wellness. For example, how do each of these components contribute to fitness and health?

• Divide the class into five groups. Assign each group to conduct research and make a short presentation on one of the components of health-related physical fitness.

SUGGESTED STUDENT ACTIVITIES

• Organize a "field trip" to a local fitness/wellness center that maintains a well-rounded program of exercise and behavior modification to promote health and fitness.

SUPPLEMENTAL READINGS

American Heart Association. Heart and Stroke Facts. Dallas, Texas. 1994.

Barrow, M. Heart talk: Understanding Cardiovascular Diseases. Cor-Ed Publishing, Gainesville, FL. 1992.

Margen, S. et al. (Eds.) The Wellness Encyclopedia. Houghton Mifflin Company, Boston, 1991.

Williams, M. Lifetime Fitness and Wellness. W. C. Brown, Dubuque, IA. 1996.

EXAM QUESTIONS

Multiple choice

1. Which of the following is not considered to be a health benefit of exercise?

    a. reduced risk of heart disease

    b. reduced risk of kidney disease

    c. reduced risk of diabetes

    d. reduced risk of bone loss with age

    Answer: b, factual, pages 4-5

2. Which of the following is not considered to be one the major components of health-related physical fitness?

    a. cardiorespiratory fitness

    b. muscular endurance

    c. body composition

    d. motor skills

Answer: d, factual, page 7

3. Total wellness can be achieved by a balance of
   a. cardiorespiratory fitness and flexibility
   b. physical, emotional, intellectual, social, and spiritual health
   c. physical, social, and mental health
   d. psychological and physical health
   Answer: b, factual, page 10

4. Exercise goal setting is considered to be
   a. unessential in a fitness program
   b. good but not required for maintenance of an exercise program
   c. a key component in the maintenance of lifetime fitness program
   d. none of above are correct
   Answer: c, factual, page 12

5. Wellness can be defined as
   a. feeling good
   b. a state of high physical fitness
   c. a state of optimal health
   d. a state of good emotional health
   Answer: c, factual, page 10

6. Another term for "heart attack" is
   a. angina
   b. fatty plaque
   c. myocardial infarction
   d. none of above are correct
   Answer: c, factual, page 5

7. Diabetes is a disease characterized by
   a. low blood sugar levels
   b. high blood glucose levels
   c. hypoglycemia
   d. none of above are correct
   Answer: b, factual, page 4

8. Muscular strength is defined as

    a. the ability of a muscle group to shorten rapidly

    b. the ability of a muscle to generate force over and over

    c. the ability of a muscle to generate low power output

    d. the maximal ability of a muscle to generate force

    Answer: d, factual, page 8

9. Muscular endurance is defined as

    a. the ability of a muscle to generate maximal force

    b. the ability of a muscle to generate force over and over again

    c. the ability of a muscle to generate high power outputs

    d. none of above are correct

    Answer: b, factual, page 8

True/False

10. Good nutrition means that an individual's diet provides all of the nutrients needed to promote growth and repair of body tissues.

    a. true

    b. false

    Answer: a, factual, page 11

11. Regular exercise can reduce your risk of heart disease.

    a. true

    b. false

    Answer: a, factual, page 4

12. The loss of bone mass and strength is called osteoporosis.

    a. true

    b. false

    Answer: a, factual, page 4

13. Regular exercise does not reduce the risk of developing type II diabetes.

    a. true

    b. false

    Answer: b, factual, page 4

14. A heart attack damages muscle cells of the heart, resulting in an impairment of the heart's ability to pump blood.
    a. true
    b. false
    Answer: a, factual, page 5

15. Coronary artery disease results from a collection of fatty material in the blood
    vessels of the heart.
    a. true
    b. false
    Answer: a, factual, page 5

16. Regular exercise can guarantee good health.
    a. true
    b. false
    Answer: b, factual, page 6

17. Regular exercise can improve longevity.
    a. true
    b. false
    Answer: a, factual, page 6

18. Improvement of motor skills is a key component of health-related physical fitness.
    a. true
    b. false
    Answer: b, factual, page 7

19. Flexibility is the ability to move joints freely through their full range of motion.
    a. true
    b. false
    Answer: a, factual, page 8

20. A lack of physical activity has been shown to play a major role in gaining body fat.
    a. true
    b. false
    Answer: a, factual, page 9

21. Physical health is defined as a freedom from disease and includes physical fitness.
    a. true
    b. false
    Answer: a, factual, page 10

22. Good nutrition plays no role in the development of physical fitness.
    a. true
    b. false
    Answer: b, page 11

DISCUSSION

23. Discuss the term "body composition". page 9

24. Define cardiorespiratory endurance. page 7

25. Define and discuss the wellness concept. pages 9-12

27. Discuss four major health benefits of regular exercise. pages 4-6

28. Discuss fitness training for sport performance vs. training for health-related fitness. pages 6- 7

29. List and discuss the five components of health-related fitness. pages 7-9

30. List the seven key points in exercise goal setting. Why are each of these components important to goal setting? page 12

31. Discuss the causes of a myocardial infarction. page 5

32. Discuss each of the five components of wellness. pages 10-12

33. Discuss the role of exercise in maintaining physical working capacity during aging. pages 4-5

Chapter 2
Fitness Evaluation-Self Testing

CHAPTER SUMMARY

1. Prior to beginning a fitness program (or performing a fitness evaluation), you should evaluate your health status.

2. An objective evaluation of your current fitness status is important before beginning an exercise training program. Further, periodic re-testing can provide feedback about your training progress.

3. Cardiorespiratory endurance is the ability of the heart to pump oxygen-rich blood to exercising muscles; this translates into the ability to perform endurance type exercise. Field tests to evaluate cardiorespiratory fitness include: 1) 1.5 mile run test; 2) 3 mile walking test; 3) submaximal cycle exercise test; and 4) step test.

4. Muscular strength is the maximum amount of force you can produce with one contraction. The most popular test to evaluate muscular strength is the one repetition maximum (1-RM) test.

5. Muscular endurance is the ability of a muscle group to generate force over and over again. Two commonly used tests of muscular endurance are the push-up and sit-up tests.

6. Flexibility is defined as the ability to move joints freely through their full range of motion. Although flexibility is joint specific, two popular tests to evaluate flexibility are the sit-an- reach test and the shoulder flexibility test.

7. Body composition is an important component of health-related physical fitness because a high percentage of body fat is associated with an increased risk of disease. In the field, the amount of body fat can be estimated using skinfold

measurements, assessment of the Body Mass Index, or examination of the waist-to-hip circumference ratio.

LEARNING OBJECTIVES

After studying this chapter, you should be able to do:

1. Explain the principle behind field-testing of cardiorespiratory fitness using the following tests:

   a) 1.5 mile run test; b) 1 mile walking test; c) cycle ergometer exercise test; and d) step test.

2. Outline the design of the one repetition maximum test for measurement of muscular strength.

3. Compare the push-up and sit-up tests as a means of evaluating muscular endurance.

4. Define the term flexibility and discuss two field tests used to assess flexibility.

5. Discuss why assessment of body composition is important in health-related fitness testing.

6. Explain how body composition is assessed using the following tests: a) hydrostatic weighting; b) skinfold test; c) Body Mass Index; and d) waist-to-hip circumference ratio.

Lecture Outline

Key Points	Subpoints	Examples
Evaluating health status prior to beginning an exercise training program	1. Need for medical exam varies as a function of age	Exercise ECG needed for males >40 years old and females >45 years

Key Points	Subpoints	Examples
Measuring cardiorespiratory fitness	1. Direct measurement of VO_2 max	
	2. Field tests	1. 1.5 mile run
		2. 1 mile walking test
		3. cycle ergometer test
		4. step test
Evaluation of muscular strength	1. 1 RM test	Bench press
		Biceps curl
		Shoulder press
		Leg press
Evaluation of muscular endurance	1. Numerous tests exist	Pushup test
		Sit-up test
Assessment of flexibility	1. Numerous tests exist	Trunk flexibility
		Shoulder flexibility
Assessment of body composition	1. Numerous techniques are available	1. Hydrostatic weighting
		2. Skinfold test
		3. Waist-to-hip circumference ratio
		4. Body mass index
		5. Height/weight tables

LAB ACTIVITIES

LABORATORY 2.1, page 43

Prior to performing any of the fitness evaluation tests, students should complete the *Health status questionnaire* (Laboratory 2-1). The objective of this laboratory is to determine if any pre-existing medical conditions warrant a medical exam prior to beginning an exercise program.

LABORATORY 2.2, page 45

Chapter two provides a series of laboratories aimed at evaluating physical fitness. Laboratories 2-2, 2-3, 2-4, and 2-5 are assessments of cardiorespiratory fitness using the 1.5 mile run, 1 mile walk, submaximal cycle test, and the step test, respectively. A wide range of cardiorespiratory labs are provided in order to allow the instructor the opportunity to choose the cardiorespiratory test that is best suited for their needs.

Laboratory 2-6 provides an opportunity to evaluate muscular strength and Laboratory 2-7 provides assessment of muscular endurance. Laboratories 2-8 and 2-9 provide opportunities to evaluate flexibility and body composition, respectively.

DISCUSSION ACTIVITIES
• Discuss the importance of regular physical fitness testing.
• Discuss the principle behind the estimation of VO_2 max by field tests (e.g. 1.5 mile run).

SUGGESTED STUDENT ACTIVITIES
• Organize a class trip to an exercise testing laboratory to observe a maximal oxygen uptake test and/or underwater weighting to determine body composition.

SUPPLEMENTAL READINGS
Getchell, B. Physical Fitness: A Way of Life. Macmillan Publishing Company, New York. 1992.

Howley, E. and B. D. Franks. Health Fitness: Instructors Handbook. Human Kinetics Publishers, Champaign, Illinois. 1992.

Williams, M. Lifetime Fitness and Wellness. W. C. Brown, Dubuque, IA. 1996.

EXAM QUESTIONS

Multiple choice

1. Performing a fitness test provides
   - a. an objective evaluation of your fitness status
   - b. you with a health-risk assessment
   - c. you with an index of your cardiac risk
   - d. none of above are correct
   - Answer: a, factual, page 19

2. An individual with an orthopedic foot problem might have difficulty performing many of the popular field tests to evaluate cardiorespiratory fitness. A field test that might be suitable for this individual is the
   - a. 1. 5 mile run
   - b. 1 mile walk test
   - c. cycle ergometer test
   - d. step test
   - Answer: c, factual, page 22

3. Muscular strength is defined as
   - a. the maximum number of repetitions that can be performed with a given weight
   - b. the maximum amount of force you can produce with one contraction
   - c. the maximum ability of a muscle group to generate force over and over again
   - d. none of above are correct
   - Answer: b, factual, page 28

4. A commonly used test of muscular endurance is
   - a. step test
   - b. 1 RM test
   - c. sit-up test
   - d. both a and b are correct
   - Answer: c, factual, page 31

5. Body composition is an important component of health-related physical fitness because
    a. a high percentage of body fat is associated with impaired muscular strength
    b. a high percentage of body fat is associated with an increased risk of disease
    c. a high percentage of body fat impairs muscular growth
    d. none of above are correct
    Answer: b, factual, page 35

6. The "gold standard" test to determine the percent of body fat of an individual is
    a. skinfold test
    b. hydrostatic weighing
    c. waist-to-hip circumference ratio
    d. body mass index
    Answer: b, factual, page 35

7. Flexibility is defined as
    a. ability to generate high muscular force
    b. agility
    c. ability to move joints freely through a full range of motion
    d. none of above is correct
    Answer: c, factual, page 33

8. The sit-and-reach test measures
    a. shoulder flexibility
    b. the ability to flex the leg muscles
    c. the ability to flex the trunk
    d. none of above are correct
    Answer: c, factual, page 34

9. Assessment of body composition by the skinfold test estimates body fat by
    a. direct measurement of total body fat
    b. measurement of subcutaneous body fat
    c. measurement of total body water
    d. both a and c are correct
    Answer: b, factual, page 35

10. Body mass index
    a. is the ratio of body weight divided by height^2
    b. is the ratio of body mass to leg length
    c. is the ratio of body mass to arm girth
    d. is the ratio of percent body fat to lean body mass
    Answer: a, factual, page 39

TRUE/FALSE

11. Males over the age of 40 years old do not need an exercise stress test prior to beginning an exercise program.
    a. true
    b. false
    Answer: b, factual, page 20

12. Cardiorespiratory endurance is a measure of the endurance capacity of both the cardiorespiratory system and exercising skeletal muscles.
    a. true
    b. false
    Answer: a, factual, page 20

13. Height and weight tables are an excellent means of estimating the ideal body weight of an individual.
    a. true
    b. false
    Answer: b, factual, page 40

14. Flexibility is defined as the ability to move joints freely through their full range of motion.
    a. true
    b. false
    Answer: a, factual, page 33

15. An exercise stress test is useful to diagnose several types of cardiovascular problems.
    a. true
    b. false

Answer: a, factual, page 20

16. The contents of a pre-exercise meal can improve performance on a fitness test.
    a. true
    b. false
    Answer: b, factual, page 21

17. A major concern with the 1-RM test is the risk of injury.
    a. true
    b. false
    Answer: a, factual, page 28

DISCUSSION

18. Describe the following field tests to evaluate cardiorespiratory fitness: 1) 1.5 mile run test; 2) 1 mile walking test; 3) cycle ergometer exercise test; and 4) step test. pages 20-27

19. Discuss the one repetition maximum (1 RM) test for measurement of muscular strength. pages 28

20. Explain how the push-up and sit-up tests are used to evaluate muscular endurance. pages 31-33

21. Discuss the concept that flexibility is joint specific. page 33-34

22. Identify two field tests to examine flexibility. pages 33-34

23. Define muscular strength. page 28

24. Discuss the skinfold test to assess body composition. pages 35-36

25. How can measurement of the waist-to-hip circumference ratio and body mass index be used to assess body composition? pages 36-39

26. Discuss the concept of VO_2 max. page 26

27. Define the term "relative VO_2 max". page 26

16

28. Why are height/weight tables not a recommended method of determining body composition? page 40

29. Discuss the concept of "optimal body composition". page 40

30. Discuss the technique of measuring heart rate using the palpation method. page 26

17

Chapter 3
General Principles of Exercise for Health and Fitness

CHAPTER SUMMARY

1. The overload principle is the most important principle of exercise training. In order to improve physical fitness, the body or muscle used during exercise must be overloaded.

2. The principle of progression states that "overload" should be increased gradually during the course of a physical fitness program.

3. The required rest period between exercise training sessions is referred to as the principle of recuperation.

4. Physical fitness can be lost due to inactivity; this is often called the principle of reversibility.

5. The components of the exercise prescription include: a) fitness goals; b) mode of exercise; c) warm-up; d) the workout; and the e) cool-down.

6. All exercise training programs need to be individualized to meet the objectives of the individual. Therefore, the exercise prescription should consider the individual's age, health, fitness status, musculoskeletal condition, and body composition.

7. The minimum dose of exercise required to improve health-related physical fitness is called the threshold of training. The minimum level of physical activity required to achieve some of the health benefits of exercise is called the threshold of health benefits.

Learning objectives

After studying this chapter, you should be able to do the following:

1. Discuss the following concepts of physical fitness: a) overload principle; b) specificity of exercise; c) principle of recuperation; and d) reversibility of training effects.

2. Outline the physiological objectives of a warm-up and cool-down.

3. Identify the general principles of exercise prescription.

4. Discuss the concepts of progression and maintenance of exercise training.

5. Explain why individualizing the workout is an important concept for the development of an exercise prescription.

6. Explain how the "threshold for health benefits" differs from the "threshold of training".

LECTURE OUTLINE

Key Points	Subpoints	Examples
Principles of training	1. Overload principle	Increasing exercise duration
	2. Progression	Overload should be gradually increased
	3. Specificity of exercise	Only exercised limbs become trained
	4. Principle of recuperation	Recovery between exercise bouts is important-failure to properly recovery can result in over-training
	5. Reversibility of training	Fitness is lost due to detraining

Key Points	Subpoints	Examples
Exercise prescription	1. Fitness goals	Every exercise prescription requires establishment of short-term and long-term fitness goals
	2. Mode of exercise	Running, cycling, swimming, etc.
	3. Warm-up	Light exercise to elevate muscle temperature and increase blood flow to muscles
	4. Primary conditioning period	Frequency, intensity, and duration of exercise
	5. Cool-down	Low intensity exercise
	6. Need to individualize the workout	Everyone differs in initial fitness status

----

LABORATORY ACTIVITIES

No laboratories are included in this chapter

DISCUSSION ACTIVITIES

• Organize a class discussion around the application of: 1) the overload principle; 2) principle of progression; 3) concept of specificity of exercise; 4) principle of recuperation; and 5) principle of recuperation.

• Invite a local training expert (e.g. well trained track coach or exercise physiologist) to class to discuss the symptoms of overtraining.

SUGGESTED STUDENT ACTIVITIES

• Require students to develop a set of 1) short-term; 2) long-term; and 3) lifetime fitness goals. Goals should be written down and should be realistic.

SUPPLEMENTAL READINGS

Getchell, B. Physical Fitness: A Way of Life. Macmillan Publishing Company, New York. 1992.

Howley, E. and B. D. Franks. Health Fitness: Instructors Handbook. Human Kinetics Publishers, Champaign, Illinois. 1992.

Williams, M. Lifetime Fitness and Wellness. Brown and Benchmark, Dubuque, IA. 1996.

EXAM QUESTIONS

Multiple choice

1. In regard to physical fitness, the overload principle can be defined as
>   a. lifting too much weight during a weight lifting procedure
>   b. overloading the body by exercise stress results in an improvement in physical fitness
>   c. overloading the body results in muscular damage
>   d. overloading tendons with excessive use results in damage
>   answer: b, factual, pages 63-64

2. The principle of progression states that
>   a. exercise overload should be increased gradually during training
>   b. an exercise training session should be followed by a recovery period
>   c. an exercise training session should progress rapidly
>   d. none of above is correct
>   answer: a, factual, page 64

3. Physical fitness can be lost due to inactivity; this is termed
>   a. the overload principle
>   b. the principle of progression
>   c. the principle of detraining
>   d. the principle of reversibility
>   answer: d, factual, page 66

4. The components of the exercise prescription include
>   a. fitness goals
>   b. mode of exercise

21

c. warm-up

d. all of above

answer: d, factual, pages 67 .

5. All exercise programs should be individualized to the individual. Therefore, the exercise prescription should consider

    a. the individual's age

    b. previous exercise habits (i.e. fitness status)

    c. health

    d. all of above

    answer: d, factual, page 70

6. The minimum dose of exercise required to improve health-related physical fitness is called

    a. the anaerobic threshold

    b. the lactate threshold

    c. the aerobic threshold

    d. none of above are correct

    answer: d, factual, page 70-71

7. Failure to get adequate rest between workouts is often defined as

    a. the general adaptation syndrome

    b. sleep apnea

    c. chronic fatigue syndrome

    d. over-training

    answer: d, factual, page 65

8. The amount of rest that is required between heavy exercise bouts is generally

    a. 4-6 hours

    b. 1-2 days

    c. 2-3 days

    d. 3-4 days

    answer: b, factual, page 65

9. A period of rest between exercise training sessions is critical for maximal improvement in physical fitness. This is often referred to as

a. the principle of progression

b. the principle of overload

c. the principle of recuperation

d. none of above are correct

answer: c, factual, page 65

True/False

10. The specificity principle refers to the fact that training is specific to those muscles exercised.

    a. true

    b. false

    answer: a, factual, page 64-65

11. The principle of progression is an extension of the overload principle.

    a. true

    b. false

    answer: a, factual, page 64

12. A period of rest between training sessions is essential to achieve optimal physical fitness.

    a. true

    b. false

    answer: a, factual, page 65

13. A diet that is inadequate in terms of the recommended amounts of carbohydrates and proteins has a limited effect on overtraining.

    a. true

    b. false

    answer: b, factual, page 66

14. After cessation of training, muscular strength is lost faster than muscular endurance.

    a. true

    b. false

    answer: b, factual, page 66

15. Exercise goals are not considered to be a part of the exercise prescription.

   a. true

   b. false

   answer: b, factual, page 67

16. The loss of fitness due to inactivity is termed the principle of reversibility.

   a. true

   b. false

   answer: a, factual, page 66

17. Every exercise prescription must include at least one mode of exercise.

   a. true

   b. false

   answer: a, factual, page 68

18. The primary purpose of a warm-up is to activate the central nervous system.

   a. true

   b. false

   answer: b, factual, page 68-69

19. The intensity of exercise is the amount of physiological stress placed on the body during exercise.

   a. true

   b. false

   answer: a, factual, page 69

20. A primary purpose of a cool-down is to return blood located in the periphery back to the heart.

   a. true

   b. false

   answer: a, factual, page 70

DISCUSSION

21. Define the following terms: over-training and principle of recuperation. page

   65

22. What is the general purpose of a cool-down and warm-up? page 70

23. Describe and discuss the components of the exercise prescription. pages 67-71

24. How does the principle of progression apply to the exercise prescription? pages 64 and 69

25. Explain why individualizing the workout is important. page 70

26. Define the "threshold for health benefits" and the "threshold of training". pages 70-71

27. What happens to physical fitness if you stop training? page 66

28. Discuss the ten percent rule. Why is this "rule" important in planning training progression? page 64

29. Discuss the symptoms of overtraining. page 65

30. Discuss the importance of goal setting in developing a physical fitness program. page 67

31. Discuss the three primary goals of a cool-down. page 70

25

Chapter 4
Exercise Prescription Guidelines: Cardiorespiratory Fitness

CHAPTER SUMMARY

1. Benefits of cardiorespiratory fitness include a lower risk of disease, feeling better, increased capacity to perform everyday tasks and improved self-esteem.

2. ATP is required for muscular contraction and can be produced in muscles by two systems: 1)anaerobic (without oxygen); and 2) aerobic (with oxygen).

3. The energy to perform many types of exercise comes from both anaerobic and aerobic sources. In general, anaerobic energy production dominates in short-term exercise whereas aerobic energy production dominates during prolonged exercise.

4. The term "cardiorespiratory system" refers to the cooperative work of the circulatory and respiratory systems. The primary function of the circulatory system is to transport blood carrying oxygen and nutrients to body tissues. The principal function of the respiratory system is to load oxygen into and remove carbon dioxide from the blood.

5. The maximum capacity to transport and utilize oxygen during exercise is called VO_2 max; VO_2 max is considered by many exercise physiologists to be the most valid measurement of cardiorespiratory fitness.

6. Cardiac output, systolic blood pressure, and heart rate increase as a function of exercise intensity. Breathing (ventilation) also increases in proportion to exercise intensity.

7. The basis for prescribing exercise to improve cardiorespiratory fitness is knowledge of the individual's initial fitness and health status.

8. Three primary elements comprise the exercise prescription: 1) warm-up; 2) workout: primary conditioning period; and 3) cool-down.

9. The purpose of a warm-up is to slowly elevate heart rate, muscle blood flow, and body temperature .

10. The components of the workout are the mode, frequency, intensity, and duration of exercise.

11. In general, the mode of exercise to be used to obtain increased cardiorespiratory endurance is one that uses a large muscle mass in a slow, rhythmical pattern for 20-60 minutes.

12. The target heart rate is the range of exercise heart rates that correspond to 50-85% of VO$_2$ max.

13. The recommended frequency of exercise to improve cardiorespiratory fitness is 3-5 times per week.

14. The purpose of a cool-down is to slowly decrease the pulse rate and return blood back to the upper body. The activity used during the training phase should be continued, but the intensity gradually decreased.

15. Establishing both short-term and long-term fitness goals is essential before beginning a fitness program.

16. Regardless of your initial fitness level, the exercise prescription to improve cardiorespiratory fitness has three phases: 1) the starter phase; 2) the slow progression phase; and 3) the maintenance phase.

17. Common endurance training techniques to improve cardiorespiratory fitness include: cross-training: long, slow distance training; interval training; and fartlek training.

18. Aerobic exercise training results in an improvement in cardiorespiratory fitness (VO$_2$ max) and muscular endurance and can result in a reduction in percent of body fat.

19. Maintaining a regular exercise routine will require proper time management and choosing physical activities that you enjoy.

LEARNING OBJECTIVES

After studying this chapter, the student should be able to:

1. Explain the benefits of developing cardiorespiratory fitness.

2. Identify the three energy systems involved in the production of ATP for muscular contraction.

3. Discuss the role of the circulatory and respiratory system during exercise.

4. Define VO$_2$ max.

5. Identify the major changes that occur in skeletal muscles, the circulatory system, and the respiratory system in response to aerobic training.

6. Explain the purpose of a warm-up.

7. List several modes of training used to improve cardiovascular fitness

8. Discuss the benefits of a cool-down at the completion of a workout.

Key Points	Subpoints	Examples
How the body adapts to exercise determines level of fitness	1. Cardiovascular function improves to deliver more O_2 to muscles	Stroke volume and cardiac output increase
	2. Respiratory muscle endurance increases	
	3. Skeletal muscles increase capacity for aerobic energy production	VO_2 max is increased
	4. Body fat is likely reduced	

LAB ACTIVITIES

LABORATORY 4.1   (Page 99)

Students should complete *Developing your personal exercise prescription* laboratory (Laboratory 4-1). The purpose of this laboratory is to allow the student to design an exercise prescription (phase, frequency, intensity, duration and mode).

LABORATORY 4.2   (Page 101)

Students should complete the *Cardiorespiratory training log* laboratory (Laboratory 4-2). The purpose of this laboratory is to allow the student to maintain a training log with the ability to monitor those factors which are essential for an exercise prescription (phase, frequency, intensity, duration and mode).

DISCUSSION ACTIVITIES

- Have a class discussion of the types of activities which would cause adaptation of the anaerobic vs. the aerobic energy systems.
- Divide the class into 4 groups. Let each group define one of four component of the exercise prescription (frequency, intensity, duration and mode) and present options for modifying each.

SUGGESTED STUDENT ACTIVITIES

- Students can visit an exercise testing lab at a local hospital or university to observe an exercise test.

30

- Have a track coach talk to the class about the ways athletes train for sports as opposed to training for fitness.

SUPPLEMENTAL READINGS

Cooper, K. The Aerobics Program for Total Well-being. M. Evans, New York, 1982.

Neiman, David C. Fitness and Sports Medicine: An introduction. Bull Publishing Co., Palo Alto, CA. 1995

Pollock, M.L. and J.H. Wilmore. 1990. *Exercise in Health and Disease.* 2nd edition. Philadelphia:W.B. Saunders.

Powers, S. and E. Howley. Exercise Physiology: Theory and Application to Fitness and Performance. 2nd Edition. W. C. Brown Publishing Co. Dubuque, Iowa. 1994.

EXAM QUESTIONS

Multiple choice

1. Which of the following are benefits of cardiorespiratory fitness?
>   a. Increased strength
>   b. Increased mental abilities
>   c. reduction in risk for heart disease
>   d. reduced risk of kidney disease
>   Answer: c, page 75, factual

2. Most of the ATP synthesized in muscle cells during aerobic exercise comes from:
>   a. stored ATP
>   b. anaerobic pathways
>   c. aerobic pathways
>   d. none of the above
>   Answer: c, page 75, factual

3. The primary anaerobic pathway for synthesizing ATP during exercise is:
>   a. Krebs cycle
>   b. beta oxidation
>   c. glycolysis
>   d. none of the above
>   Answer: b, page 76, factual

4. A problem in the anaerobic synthesis of energy is that a by-product of glycolysis is the formation of:

   a. fat

   b. carbon dioxide

   c. water

   d. lactic acid

   Answer: d, page 76, conceptual

5. Which of the following describes the pathway for blood flow through the systemic circulation?

   a. veins - capillaries - arteries

   b. arteries - capillaries - veins

   c. capillaries - veins - arteries

   d. veins - arteries - capillaries

   Answer: b, page 78, conceptual

6. Which of the following is used to calculate maximal exercise heart rate.

   a. 200 + age

   b. 220 - age

   c. 200 + 85% of age

   d. none of the above

   Answer: b, page 79, factual

7. The highest blood pressure which is reached during the contraction phase of the heart cycle is:

   a. diastolic

   b. stroke volume

   c. systolic

   d. pulmonary

   Answer: c, page 79, factual

8. Approximately what percentage of adults in the U.S. are hypertensive?

   a. 20

   b. 40

   c. 60

d. 80

Answer: a, page 80, factual

9. Normal blood pressure for a college-aged male is approximately:

    a. 100/80

    b. 100/60

    c. 120/100

    d. 120/80

    Answer: d, page 80, factual

10. The anaerobic threshold refers to the point during aerobic exercise at which:

    a. breathing is maximal

    b. heart rate is maximal

    c. there is an increased rate of lactic acid accumulation

    d. breathing has returned to normal

    Answer: c, page 82, conceptual

11. Breathing increases during exercise to:

    a. bring in more oxygen

    b. remove carbon dioxide

    c. both of these

    d. none of these

    Answer; c, page 81, factual

12. The primary components of an exercise prescription to improve cardiovascular fitness includes:

    a. mode

    b. anaerobic threshold

    c. VO2 max

    d. Systole

    Answer: a, page 83, factual

13. Which of the following adaptations occurs with exercise training?

    a. exercise stroke volume decreases

    b. exercise cardiac output decreases

    c. VO2 max increases

d. skeletal muscles significantly increase strength

Answer: c, page 92, conceptual

14. Which of the following refers to a training technique utilizing several different modes of training?

a. Fartlek

b. Cross training

c. Long, slow distance

d. Interval training

Answer: b, page 90, factual

15. Which of the following modes of exercise is considered the best for achieving cardiorespiratory fitness?

a. cycling

b. stretching

c. calisthenics

d. weight lifting

Answer: a, page 83, factual

TRUE / FALSE

16. Increased strength and reduced risk of kidney disease are benefits of cardiorespiratory fitness.

a. True

b. False

Answer: b, page 76, factual

17. Energy is stored in muscles cells as lactic acid.

a. True

b. False

Answer: b, page 76, factual

18. Energy to perform prolonged, endurance exercise is produced from the anaerobic energy system.

a. True

b. False

Answer: b, page 76, factual

19. Stroke volume is the amount of blood pumped by the heart with each beat.
    a. True
    b. False
    Answer: a, page 78, factual

20. Arteries carry blood away from the heart.
    a. True
    b. False
    Answer: a, page 78, factual

21. Cardiac output is the product of heart rate times stroke volume
    a. True
    b. False
    Answer: a, page 78, factual

22. VO_2 max is the maximal amount of exercise that can be performed by an individual.
    a. True
    b. False
    Answer: b, page 80, factual

23. Systolic blood pressure is the pressure in the arterial system during the contraction phase of the heart.
    a. True
    b. False
    Answer: a, page 79, factual

24. The heart rate which corresponds to an exercise intensity sufficient to improve fitness is called the target heart rate.
    a. True
    b. False
    Answer: a, page 84, factual

25. Only one mode of exercise is recommended for increasing cardiorespiratory fitness.
   a. True
   b. False
   Answer: b, page 83, conceptual

26. The duration of an exercise session refers to the number of times per week that exercise is performed.
   a. True
   b. False
   Answer: b, page 84, factual

27. A cool-down is defined as 5-15 minutes of light exercises and stretching.
   a. True
   b. False
   Answer: a, page 86, factual

28. The slow progression phase of an exercise program refers to the intensity and duration of workout that is maintained for life.
   a. True
   b. False
   Answer: b, page 88, factual

29. Cross-training refers to training that utilizes various modes of exercise to improve cardiorespiratory fitness.
   a. True
   b. False
   Answer: a, page 90, factual

30. Long, slow distance training requires a steady, submaximal exercise intensity.
   a. True
   b. False
   Answer: a, page 91, factual

31. Endurance training results in an increase in maximal stroke volume.
   a. True

b. False

Answer: a, page 92, conceptual

32. Endurance training results in an increase in VO_2 max.

   a. True
   b. False

   Answer: a, page 93, conceptual

DISCUSSION

33. Discuss the two systems which produce energy during exercise and the conditions under which each predominates.

   Answer: page 76, conceptual

34. What two factors determine cardiac output and how are they changed during exercise.

   Answer: page 78, conceptual

35. Define hypertension?

   Answer: page 80, conceptual

36. Why should a warm-up be performed before a workout?

   Answer: page 82, conceptual

37. Discuss the components of an exercise prescription to improve cardiorespiratory fitness.

   Answer: page 83, conceptual

38. How is maximal heart rate determined?

   Answer: page 84, conceptual

39. What is the range of exercise intensity necessary to improve cardiorespiratory fitness?

   Answer: page 84, conceptual

41. What is the purpose of the maintenance phase of an exercise program?
    Answer: page 88, conceptual

42. What endurance training techniques are recommended for improving cardiorespiratory fitness?
    Answer: page 90, conceptual

43. What factors determine how much VO2 max will increase after an endurance training program?
    Answer: page 93, conceptual

Chapter 5
Improving Muscular Strength and Endurance

CHAPTER SUMMARY

1. The importance of training to improve strength and endurance is evident from the fact that strength training can reduce low-back pain, reduce the incidence of exercise related injuries, decrease the incidence of osteoporosis, and aid in maintenance of functional capacity which normally decreases with age.

2. Muscular strength is defined as the ability of a muscle to generate maximal force (see Chapter 1).   In simple terms, this means how much weight that an individual can lift during one maximal effort. In contrast, muscular endurance is defined as the ability of a muscle to generate force over and over again. In general, increasing muscular strength by exercise training will increase muscular endurance as well. In contrast, training aimed at improving muscular endurance does not always result in significant improvements in muscular strength.

3. Skeletal muscle is composed of a collection of long thin cells (called fibers).   Muscles are attached to bone by thick connective tissue known as tendons. Therefore muscular contraction results in the tendons pulling on bone and thereby causing movement.

4. Muscle contraction is regulated by signals coming from motor nerves. Motor nerves originate in the spinal cord and send nerve fibers to individual muscles throughout the body. The motor nerve and all the muscle fibers it controls is called a motor unit.

5. Muscle contraction occurs as a result of the interaction of two contractile proteins (actin and myosin). The "sliding filament theory" of muscular contraction proposes that muscular shortening occurs as a result of actin sliding over the myosin.

6. Isotonic or dynamic contractions are contractions that result in movement of a body part. Isometric contractions involve the development of force but results in no movement of body parts. Concentric contractions are isotonic muscle contractions involving muscle shortening. In contrast, eccentric contractions

(also called negative contractions) are defined as isotonic contractions in which the muscle exerts force while the muscle lengthens.

7. Human skeletal muscle can be classified into three major fiber types: 1) slow twitch; 2) intermediate; and 3) fast twitch fibers. Slow twitch fibers shorten slowly but are highly fatigue resistant. Fast twitch fibers shorten rapidly but fatigue rapidly. Intermediate fibers possess a combination of the characteristics of fast and slow twitch fibers.

8. The process of involving more muscle fibers to produce increased muscular force is called *fiber recruitment*.

9. The percentage of slow, intermediate, and fast-twitch fibers varies among individuals. Research by sports scientists has shown that a relationship exists between muscle fiber type and success in athletics. For example, champion endurance athletes (e.g. marathon runners) have a high percentage of slow-twitch fibers.

10. There are two primary physiological factors that determine the amount of force which can be generated by a muscle: 1) size of the muscle and the 2) neural influences (i.e. number of fibers recruited).

11. Muscle size is increased primarily because of an increase in fiber size (called hypertrophy). Further, recent research has shown that strength training can also promote the formation of new muscle fibers (called hyperplasia).

12. The overload principle states that a muscle will increase in strength and/or endurance only when it works against a workload which is greater than normal.

13. The concept of progressive resistance exercise (PRE) is the application of the overload principle to strength and endurance exercise programs.

14. A weight training program using low repetitions/high resistance results in the greatest strength gains whereas a weight training program using high repetitions/low resistance results in the greatest improvement in muscular endurance.

15. Isotonic programs, like an isotonic contraction, utilize the concept of contracting a muscle against a moveable load (usually a free weight or weights mounted by cables or chains to form a weight "machine"). An isometric strength training program is based on the concept of contracting a muscle(s) at a fixed angle against an immovable object (isometric or static contraction). Isokinetic

exercises require the use of machines that govern the speed of movement during muscle contraction throughout the range of motion.

16. To begin a strength training program, divide the program into 3 phases: Initial Phase -- 2-3 weeks / 2 workouts per week / 2 sets / 15 RM; Progression Phase -- 20 weeks / 2-3 workouts per week / 3 sets / 6 RM; Maintenance Phase -- Continues for life / 1 workout per week / 3 sets / 6 RM.

LEARNING OBJECTIVES

After studying this chapter, the student should be able to:

1. Explain the benefits of developing muscular strength and endurance.
2. Describe how muscles contract.
3. Distinguish between the various types of muscle fibers.
4. Classify the types of muscular contractions.
5. Identify the major changes that occur in skeletal muscles in response to strength training.
6. List the factors that determine muscle strength and endurance.
7. Outline the general principles used in designing a strength and endurance program.
8. Distinguish between the various types of training programs for improving strength and endurance.
9. Design a program for improving strength and endurance.

LECTURE OUTLINE

Key Points	Subpoints	Examples
Benefits of muscular strength and endurance	1. Reduce injuries	
	2. Reduce back pain	
	3. Reduce age-related decreases in strength and bone loss	Reduces osteoporosis
	4. Improves self-esteem	
	5. Increases resting energy	Muscle uses more energy than fat expenditure
Physiological basis for strength and endurance	1. Structure of muscle	Motor unit, muscle fiber, myofibril
	2. Type of contraction	Isotonic, isometric (concentric and eccentric) and isokinetic

41

Key Points	Subpoints	Examples
	3. Fiber type	Slow-, intermediate-, and fast-twitch
	4. Recruitment pattern	Slow first, then intermediate and fast
Principles of a strength and training endurance training program	1. Progressive Resistance Exercise (PRE)	Overload applied to strength
	2. Specificity	Work only muscles to be trained
Designing a strength program	1. Stress safety	See page 114 for tips
	2. High weight - low repetition	
	3. Choose isotonic, isometric or isokinetic	Isotonic most popular
Exercise Prescription for weight training	1. Intensity	Number of RM's (6-8 for strength and 18-20 for endurance)
	2. Duration	Number of sets (2-3 for strength and 4-6 for endurance)
	3. Frequency	Number of days / week (2-3)
Starting and maintaining a program	1. Starter phase	1-3 weeks
	2. Slow progression	4-20 weeks
	3. Maintenance	20+ weeks
Adaptations to strength training	1. Physiological changes	Increased muscle size (hypertrophy), increased number of fibers recruited, increased flexibility, decreased body fat.
	2. Rate of improvement	See figure 5.11 & 5.12
	3. Gender differences	See figure 5.13

LAB ACTIVITIES

LABORATORY 5.1   (Page 131)
Students should complete the *Strength Training Log* laboratory (Laboratory 5.1). The purpose of this lab is to provide a record of progress in building strength in the upper and lower body.

DISCUSSION ACTIVITIES
- Have a class discussion on the benefits of increasing muscular strength and/or endurance. Is it necessary for good health?
- Have students trace the development of strength during a strength training program (neural component, muscle component). How does the muscle adapt to cause an increase in strength?
- Divide the class into 3 groups. Assign each group one of the three types of muscle contractions and debate the pros and cons of each.
- Discuss the role of nutrition during a strength training program.
- Discuss the role of the different fiber types in determining muscle function.
- Discuss the role of anabolic steroids in weight training and the significance of the side effects.

SUGGESTED STUDENT ACTIVITIES
- Have a body builder talk to the class about the use of steroids in the gym.
- Have a strength coach talk to the class about competitive strength training versus training for fitness.

SUPPLEMENTAL READINGS
Bouchard, C., R. Shephard, T. Stephens, J. Sutton, and B. McPherson (Eds.). 1990. *Exercise, Fitness, and Health: A Consensus of Current Knowledge*. Human Kinetics Books, Champaign, IL.

Fleck, S.J. and W.J. Kraemer. 1987. Designing Resistance Training Programs. Champaign, IL, Human Kinetics Books.

Komi, P. *Strength and Power in Sport*. Blackwell Publishers, Oxford, 1992.

Powers, S. and E. Howley. 1994. *Exercise Physiology: Theory and Application to Fitness and Performance*. 2nd Edition. Brown and Benchmark Publishing Co. Dubuque, IA

d. diet
Answer: c, page 112, conceptual

14. As strength and endurance are increased with weight training, the load against
    which the muscle works must be periodically elevated for strength and
    endurance gains to be realized. This is referred to as:
    a. principle of specificity
    b. repetitions max
    c. maximal anaerobic capacity
    d. progressive resistance exercise
    Answer: d, page 112, conceptual

15. The fact that muscle strength and endurance are realized only in the muscles
    trained is referred to as:
    a. specificity
    b. recruitment
    c. overload
    d. PRE
    Answer: a, page 110, conceptual

16. Synthetic forms of the male hormone testosterone that are used to cause muscle
    hypertrophy are called:
    a. growth hormone
    b. protein powder
    c. anabolic steroids
    d. ginseng
    Answer: c, page 113, factual

17. Which of the following are safety concerns when weight training?
    a. breath-holding while lifting
    b. duration of a training session
    c. talking during a training session
    d. support belts
    Answer: a, page 114, factual

18. Which of the following should be the general rule to follow to increase endurance
    in a weight training program?
    a. high resistance - high repetitions
    b. high resistance - low repetitions
    c. low resistance - high repetitions
    d. low resistance - low repetitions
    Answer: c, page 114, conceptual

19. Which of the following should be the general rule to follow to increase strength in a
    weight training program?
    a. high resistance - high repetitions
    b. high resistance - low repetitions
    c. low resistance - high repetitions
    d. low resistance - low repetitions

46

Answer: b, page 114, conceptual

20. The intensity of exercise in a weight training program is measured by:
    a. heart rate
    b. repetition maximum
    c. perceived effort
    d. the size of the individual
    Answer: b, page 116, conceptual

21. The number of times an exercise is performed in weight training is referred to as a:
    a. repetition maximum
    b. set
    c. load
    d. taper
    Answer: b, page 116, factual

22. The phase of a weight training program in which most of the strength gains are realized is the:
    a. slow progression phase
    b. maintenance phase
    c. recruitment phase
    d. starter phase
    Answer: a, page 117, factual

23. The increase in muscle size due to weight training is called:
    a. hypertrophy
    b. hyperplasia
    c. atrophy
    d. dystrophy
    Answer: a, page 125, factual

24. The initial increase in strength seen with weight training is primarily due to:
    a. hypertrophy
    b. hyperplasia
    c. increased fiber recruitment
    d. body weight gain
    Answer: c, page 125, factual

TRUE / FALSE

25. A regular strength training program increases VO2 max.
    a. True
    b. False
    Answer: b, page 105, conceptual

26. A regular strength training program reduces resting metabolic rate.
    a. True
    b. False
    Answer: b, page 106, conceptual

27. Muscular strength is defined as the maximal weight an individual can lift in one set.
    a. True
    b. False
    Answer: b, page 106, factual

28. Muscle are attached to bones by tendons.
    a. True
    b. False
    Answer: a, page 106, factual

29. A motor nerve and all the fibers it controls is called a muscle fascia.
    a. True
    b. False
    Answer: b, page 106, conceptual

30. An isotonic contraction refers to a static contraction against an immovable object.
    a. True
    b. False
    Answer: b, page 107, conceptual

31. An isometric contraction refers to a muscle contraction against a movable object at a fixed speed.
    a. True
    b. False
    Answer: b, page 107, conceptual

32. An eccentric muscle contraction occurs when a muscle contracts while it lengthens.
    a. True
    b. False
    Answer: a, page 110, conceptual

33. A slow twitch muscle fiber contracts slowly and fatigues easily.
    a. True
    b. False
    Answer: b, page 110, conceptual

34. An intermediate twitch muscle fiber produces force quickly and also fatigues quickly.
    a. True
    b. False
    Answer: b, page 110, conceptual

35. Muscle fiber recruitment refers to the process of muscle fiber filaments sliding over each other.
    a. True
    b. False
    Answer: b, page 110, conceptual

36. Genetics is the primary determinant of muscle fiber type.
    a. True
    b. False
    Answer: a, page 111, conceptual

37. The primary determinant of how much force can be generated by muscle is muscle size.
    a. True
    b. False
    Answer: a, page 112, conceptual

38. Increasing the work load throughout a strength training program is referred to as progressive resistance exercise.
    a. True
    b. False
    Answer: a, page 112, conceptual

39. The principle of specificity refers to the notion that strength gains are made in several muscle groups surrounding those that are used during training.
    a. True
    b. False
    Answer: b, page 112, conceptual

40. Anabolic steroids are used by athletes to increase performance in endurance events such as the marathon.
    a. True
    b. False
    Answer: b, page 113, conceptual

41. Spotters are important in assisting lifting when using free weights.
    a. True
    b. False
    Answer: a, page 114, factual

42. High resistance and high repetitions should be used for optimal increase in strength in a weight training program.
    a. True
    b. False
    Answer: b, page 114, conceptual

43. Low resistance and high repetitions should be used for optimal increase in endurance in a weight training program.
    a. True
    b. False
    Answer: a, page 114, conceptual

44. Repetition maximum is the determinant of intensity of exercise in weight training.
    a. True

b. False
Answer: a, page 116, conceptual

45. The starter phase of a weight training program is the phase in which most of the weight gains are made.
    a. True
    b. False
Answer: b, page 117, factual

46. Hypertrophy is the increase in muscle fiber number seen with weight training.
    a. True
    b. False
Answer: b, page 125, factual

47. The initial increase in strength seen with weight training is primarily due to muscle hypertrophy.
    a. True
    b. False
Answer: b, page 125, factual

48. Men increase strength faster and to a greater extent than do women on similar weight training programs.
    a. True
    b. False
Answer: b, page 125, factual

DISCUSSION
49. Discuss the health benefits of strength training.
    Answer: Page 105, conceptual

50. Discuss the difference in muscle strength and muscle endurance.
    Answer: Page 106, factual

51. List the various parts of muscles and tell their functions.
    Answer: Page 106, factual

52. Discuss the function of a motor unit in a muscle contraction.
    Answer: Page 106, conceptual

53. Discuss the types of muscle contractions.
    Answer: Page 107-110, conceptual

54. Discuss the sliding filament theory of muscle contraction.
    Answer: Page 107, conceptual

55. List the three muscle fiber types and the contractile characteristics of each.
    Answer: Page 110, conceptual

56. Discuss muscle fiber recruitment in the process of generating increased amounts of force.
    Answer: Page 111, conceptual

57. What is the role of genetics and training in determining muscle fiber type.
    Answer: Page 111, conceptual

58. What factors determine strength and what is the relative role of each.
    Answer: Page 112, conceptual

59. Compare and contrast the concepts of progressive resistance exercise (PRE) and the overload principle.
    Answer: Page 112, conceptual

60. What is the principle of specificity and how should it be used during a weight training program.
    Answer: Page 112, conceptual

61. Discuss the use of anabolic steroids by athletes and bodybuilders and their side-effects.
    Answer: Page 113, conceptual

62. Discuss the design of a weight training program to optimize endurance.
    Answer: Page 114, conceptual

63. Discuss the way exercise intensity is determined in weight training.
    Answer: Page 116, conceptual

64. How is exercise duration determined in a weight training program?
    Answer: Page 114, conceptual

65. What is the recommended exercise frequency for weight training?
    Answer: Page 114, conceptual

66. List the three phases of a weight training program and describe the length of each.
    Answer: Page 116, factual

67. What is the difference in hypertrophy and hyperplasia?
    Answer: Page 125, factual

68. Discuss the time course of strength increases seen in a weight training program. What physiological changes take place that affect this adaptation?
    Answer: Page 125, factual

51

Chapter 6
Improving Flexibility

CHAPTER SUMMARY

1. Flexibility is defined as the range of motion of a joint .

2. Improved flexibility results in the following benefits: increased joint mobility, resistance to muscle injury, prevention of low-back problems, efficient body movement, and improved posture and personal appearance.

3. The structural and physiological limits to flexibility are: 1) bone, 2) muscle, 3) structures within the joint capsule, 4) the tendons which connect muscle to bones and connective tissue surrounding joints, and 5) skin.

4. If muscle spindles are suddenly stretched, they respond by producing a stretch reflex. However, if the muscles and tendons are stretched slowly, the stretch reflex can be avoided.

5. Static stretches involve stretching a muscle to the limitation of movement and holding it for an extended period of time.

6. Proprioceptive neuromuscular facilitation (PNF), combines stretching with alternating contracting and relaxing of muscles to improve flexibility.

LEARNING OBJECTIVES

After studying this chapter, the student should be able to:

1. Discuss the value of flexibility.

2. Identify the structural and physiological limits to flexibility.

3. Discuss the stretch reflex.

4. Describe the three categories of stretching techniques.

5. Design a flexibility exercise program.

LECTURE OUTLINE

Key Points	Subpoints	Examples
Benefits of Flexibility	1. Increased joint mobility 2. Resistance to muscle injury 3. Prevention of low-back pain 4. Efficient body movement 5. Good posture	
Physiological basis for developing flexibility	1. Tissues which restrict movement 2. Stretch reflex	Bone, muscle, ligaments, cartilage, tendons, and skin Muscle spindles initiate (physician tapsbelow the knee with a rubber hammer elicits quadriceps contraction)
Designing a flexibility program	1. Static 2. Proprioceptive neuromuscular	Slow movements to the point of limitation held for 20-30 sec for 3-4 times. Combines static stretching with alternating contracting and relaxing of muscles (Can be CR stretching or CRAC)
Exercise prescription for improving flexibility	1. Frequency 2. Duration 3. Intensity 4. Avoid hazardous exercises	2-5 days per week 10-30 minutes per day 20-30 seconds per stretch / 3 stretches Breath-holding, full flexion of the neck,full extension of knees-neck-back, loose joints, forceful extension or flexion of the spine

LAB ACTIVITIES

LABORATORY 6.1 (PAGE 151)
Students should complete the *Flexibility Progression Log* laboratory (Laboratory 6.1). The purpose of this log is to provide a record of progress in increasing flexibility in selected joints.

DISCUSSION ACTIVITIES
- Have a class discussion on the benefits of increasing flexibility. Is it necessary for good health?
- Divide the class into two groups and have a competition to see which group can design the greatest number of PNF stretches.

SUGGESTED STUDENT ACTIVITIES
- Have a physical therapist speak to the class about the importance of flexibility and present some common stretching exercises.
- Have a sports trainer talk to the class about how athletes utilize different stretches for different sports.

SUPPLEMENTAL READINGS
DeVries, H. and T. Housh. *Physiology of Exercise*. Fifth Edition. Brown and Benchmark. Dubuque, IA. 1994.

Fox, E., R. Bowers, and M. Foss. *The Physiological Basis for Exercise and Sports*. 5th Ed. Brown & Benchmark, Inc., Dubuque, IA, 1993.

Howley, E. and D. Franks. *Health Fitness Instructors Handbook*. Human Kinetics, Champaign, Illinois. 1992.

Hutton, R.S. Neuromuscular Basis of Stretching Exercises. In: *Strength and Power in Sport*. (ed.) Komi, P.V. Blackwell Scientific Publications, Oxford, England, 1992.

Powers, S. and E. Howley. *Exercise Physiology: Theory and Application to Fitness and Performance*. 2nd Edition. W. C. Brown Publishing Co. Dubuque, Iowa. 1994.

Sady, S.P., M. Wortman, & D. Blanke. Flexibility training: Ballistic, Static or Proprioceptive Neuromuscular Facilitation? *Archives of Physical Medicine and Rehabilitation*. 63: 261-263, 1982.

Steiner, M. E. Hypermobility and Knee Injuries. *Physician and Sports Medicine* 15: 159-168, 1987.

Wallin, D., B. Ekblom, R. Grahn, and T. Nordenborg. Improvement of Muscle Flexibility. A comparison between two techniques. *American Journal of Sports Medicine.* 13: 263-268, 1985.

EXAM QUESTIONS

MULTIPLE CHOICE

1. The ability to move joints freely through their full range of motion is referred to as:
    a. recruitment
    b. flexibility
    c. mobilization
    d. loose joints
    Answer: b, page 135, factual

2. Which of the following would be considered a benefit of increased flexibility:
    a. increased strength
    b. increased endurance
    c. resistance to muscle injury
    d. higher VO2 max
    Answer: c, page 135, factual

3. Which of the following are determinants of joint range of motion?
    a. muscle and tendons
    b. number of motor units
    c. fiber type
    d. length of bones
    Answer: a, page 136, factual

4. Which of the following is altered in a program to increase flexibility?
    a. bone
    b. cartilage
    c. tendons
    d. ligaments
    Answer: c, page 136, conceptual

5. Special muscle receptors that sense stretch are referred to as:
    a. motor units
    b. muscle fascia
    c. muscle units
    d. muscle spindles
    Answer: d, page 136, factual

6. The reaction which occurs when a muscle is suddenly stretched and stimulates muscle spindles is called a(n);
    a. stretch reflex
    b. fiber typing

c. muscle twitch
d. muscle spasm
Answer: a, page 136, conceptual

7. Stretching by slowly lengthening the muscle to a point where further movement is limited and holding that position for a fixed period of time is referred to as:
a. ballistic stretching
b. static stretching
c. CR stretching
d. CRAC stretching
Answer: b, page 136, conceptual

8. A slow stretch combined with alternating contracting and relaxing muscles is called:
a. ballistic stretching
b. static stretching
c. PNF stretching
d. passive stretching
Answer: c, page 137, conceptual

9. A very fast, bouncing type of stretch that is likely to stimulate stretch receptors and cause a stretch reflex is:
a. ballistic stretching
b. static stretching
c. PNF stretching
d. passive stretching
Answer: a, page 137, conceptual

10. To improve flexibility, stretching exercises should be performed:
a. 1 day per week
b. 2-5 days per week
c. 4-7 days per week
d. 1-3 days per week
Answer: b, page 138, factual

11. To improve flexibility, the duration of a stretching session should be:
a. 5 min
b. 10-30 min
c. 30-50 min
d. until pain is maximal
Answer: b, page 138, factual

12. The intensity of stretching is monitored by feel. In general, the limb should not be stretched beyond a position creating:
a. intense pain
b. mild discomfort
c. no sense of limitation of movement
d. normal movements
Answer: b, page 139, factual

13. Which of the following principles should be avoided in any stretching routine.
    a. flexion of the hip
    b. extension of the hip
    c. flexion of the knee or neck
    d. rotation of the trunk
    Answer: c, page 139, conceptual

TRUE / FALSE
14. Flexibility is the ability to move joints freely through their full range of motion.
    a. True
    b. False
    Answer: a, page 135, factual

15. Increased resistance to muscle injury is a benefit of increased flexibility.
    a. True
    b. False
    Answer: a, page 135, factual

16. Prevention of low-back pain is a benefit of increased flexibility.
    a. True
    b. False
    Answer: a, page 135, factual

17. Increased joint mobility is a benefit of increased flexibility.
    a. True
    b. False
    Answer: a, page 135, factual

18. Tendons are one of the contributors to limiting range of motion in a joint.
    a. True
    b. False
    Answer: a, page 136, factual

19. Skin is one of the contributors to limiting range of motion in a joint.
    a. True
    b. False
    Answer: a, page 136, factual

20. Ligaments are one of the contributors to limiting range of motion in a joint.
    a. True
    b. False
    Answer: a, page 136, factual

21. Cartilage is altered to improve flexibility in a program of regular stretching.
    a. True
    b. False
    Answer: b, page 136, factual

22. Ligaments are altered to improve flexibility in a program of regular stretching.
    a. True
    b. False
    Answer: b, page 136, factual

23. Muscle is altered to improve flexibility in a program of regular stretching.
    a. True
    b. False
    Answer: a, page 136, factual

24. Muscle spindles sense load on a muscle and a reflex relaxation.
    a. True
    b. False
    Answer: b, page 136, conceptual

25. A stretch reflex occurs when a muscle is suddenly stretched causing stimulation of muscle spindles.
    a. True
    b. False
    Answer: a, page 136, factual

26. Static stretching is achieved by slowly lengthening the muscle to a point where further movement is limited and holding that position for a fixed period of time.
    a. True
    b. False
    Answer: a, page 136, factual

27. Proprioceptive neuromuscular facilitation refers to a method of stretching which utilizes a passive stretch performed by your partner.
    a. True
    b. False
    Answer: b, page 137, factual

28. Ballistic stretches are recommended over other types of stretches because of the safety and validity of this type of stretching.
    a. True

b. False

Answer: b, page 137, conceptual

29. To improve flexibility, it is necessary to perform stretching exercises every day.
    a. True
    b. False

    Answer: b, page 138, factual

30. The duration of a stretching session for improving flexibility should last from 30 -
    50 min.
    a. True
    b. False

    Answer: b, page 138, factual

31. If stretching to improve flexibility is to be beneficial, it should incorporate exercises
    that cause some pain.
    a. True
    b. False
    Answer: b, page 139, conceptual

32. Flexion of the hip should be avoided because of the excess pressure caused in
    the abdominal area.
    a. True
    b. False
    Answer: b, page 139, conceptual

33. Forceful extension of the spine is recommended to stretch abdominal muscles.
    a. True
    b. False
    Answer: b, page 139, conceptual

DISCUSSION

34. Discuss the benefits of increased flexibility.
    Answer: Page 135, factual

35. List the anatomical factors which limit range of motion in a joint and tell which can
    be altered with a program of stretching.
    Answer: Page 136, factual

36. Define a muscle spindle and tell its importance in muscle function.
    Answer: Page 136, conceptual

59

37. What is a stretch reflex and how does it affect flexibility exercises?
    Answer: Page 136, conceptual

38. Discuss the pros and cons of the 3 types of stretching techniques.
    Answer: Page 136-7, conceptual

39. Compare CR and CRAC stretching. What is the physiological reasoning behind the CRAC method?
    Answer: Page 137, conceptual

40. Discuss the frequency, intensity and duration of stretching to improve flexibility.
    Answer: Page 138, factual

41. How is the intensity of stretching exercise determined?
    Answer: Page 139, factual

42. Discuss those considerations necessary to prevent injury in a stretching program.
    Answer: P 139, factual

Chapter 7
Nutrition, Health, and Fitness

CHAPTER SUMMARY

1. Nutrition is the study of food and its relationship to health and disease. The primary problem in nutrition in industrialized countries today is over-eating.

2. A well-balanced diet is composed of approximately 55-60% complex carbohydrates, 25-30% fat, and 12-15% protein. These macronutrients are also called the fuel nutrients, because they are the only substances that can be used as fuel and, therefore, provide the energy (calories) necessary for bodily functions.

3. Carbohydrate is a primary fuel used by the body to provide energy. The calorie is a unit of measure of the energy value of food or the energy required for physical activity.

4. Simple carbohydrates consist of sugar (glucose, fructose, sucrose) and double sugar units (galactose, lactose, and maltose).

5. The complex carbohydrates consist of the starches and fiber. Starches are composed of chains of simple sugars. Fiber is a non-digestible but essential form of complex carbohydrates (contained in whole grains, vegetables, and fruits).

6. Fat is an efficient storage form for energy, since each gram contains over twice the energy content of either carbohydrate or protein. Fat can be derived from dietary sources, and it can be formed from excess carbohydrate and protein consumed in the diet. Excess fat in the diet is stored as fat in the adipose tissues located under the skin and around internal organs. Fats are classified as either simple, compound or derived fats. The triglycerides are the most notable of the simple fats. Fatty acids are classified as either "saturated" or "unsaturated" depending on their chemical structure. For nutritional considerations, the most important of the compound fats are the lipoproteins. Cholesterol is the best example of the class of fats called derived fats.

7. The primary role of protein consumed in the diet is to serve as the structural unit to build and repair cells in all tissues of the body. Protein consists of amino acids made by the body (eleven nonessential amino acids) and those available only through dietary sources (nine essential amino acids).

8. Vitamins serve many important functions in the body including regulation of growth and metabolism. The class of water soluble vitamins consists of several B complex vitamins and vitamin C. The fat soluble vitamins are A, D, E, and K.

9. Minerals are chemical elements contained in many foods. Like vitamins, minerals serve many important roles in regulating body functions .

10. Approximately 60% of the body is water. Water is involved in all vital processes in the body and is the nutrient of greatest concern to the physically active individual. In addition to the water contained in foods, it is recommended that an additional 8 glasses of fluids should be consumed daily.

11. The basic goals of developing good nutritional habits are to maintain ideal body weight, eat a variety of foods following the "eating right pyramid" model, avoid consuming too much fat, saturated fat, and cholesterol, eat foods with adequate starch and fiber, avoid consuming too much simple sugar, avoid consuming too much sodium, and if you drink alcohol, do so in moderation.

12. The general rule for meeting the body's need for macronutrients is that an individual should consume approximately 55-60% of needed calories in carbohydrates (50% complex carbohydrates and 10% simple sugars), 25-30% or less in fats (approximately 10% saturated and 20% unsaturated fats), and 12-15% in proteins.

13. The calorie is a unit of measure of the energy value of food or the energy required for physical activity.

14. In order to have a healthy diet, several nutrients should be minimized. These are: fats (especially saturated or animal fats), cholesterol, salt, sugar/corn syrup and alcohol.

15. The intensity of exercise dictates the relative proportions of fat and carbohydrate that are consumed as fuel during exercise. In general, the lower the intensity of exercise, the more fat is used as a fuel. Conversely, the greater the intensity of exercise, the more carbohydrate is used as a fuel.

16. Antioxidants are nutrients that prevent oxygen free radicals from combining with cells and damaging them. To date, several micronutrients have been identified as potent antioxidants. These are vitamins E and C, beta-carotene, zinc, and selenium.

17. Food storage and preparation is key to preventing food poisoning. Select foods that appear clean and fresh; keep foods cold or frozen to prevent bacteria from

growing; thoroughly clean fresh fruits, vegetables and meats (especially chicken); cook all meats thoroughly; order well done meats when dining out.

LEARNING OBJECTIVES

After studying this chapter, the student should be able to:

1. Define macro- and micronutrients.
2. Describe the macronutrients and primary functions of each.
3. Discuss the energy content of fats, carbohydrates and proteins in the body.
4. Describe the micronutrients and the primary functions of each.
5. Discuss the value of water in the diet.
6. List the dietary guidelines for a well-balanced diet.
7. Define the term calorie.
8. Describe the need for protein, carbohydrate, and vitamins for physically active individuals.

LECTURE OUTLINE

Key Points	Subpoints	Examples
Basic concepts of nutrition	1. Macronutrients	The fuel nutrients - carbohydrates (simple and complex), fat (simple-compound- derived), and protein (complete-incomplete)
	2. Micronutrients	Vitamins (fat and water soluble; see table 7.5), minerals (see table 7.6) and water.
Guidelines for a healthy diet	1. Optimize nutrients	58% of calories - complex carbohydrates30% of calories - fat (10% saturated - 20% unsaturated)
	2. Reduce calories	Reduce simple sugars and fat (carbohydrate = 4 kcal/g; protein = 4 kcal/g; fat = 9 kcal/g)
	3. Perform dietary analysis	Use a 3-day recall (see Lab 7.1)
	4. Avoid foods with little nutritive value	Fat, cholesterol, salt, simple sugars, alcohol (see Figure 7.6)

Key Points	Subpoints	Examples
Nutrition and Fitness	1. Carbohydrates	People engaged in regular exercise should increase carbohydrate intake to 70% of the total caloric intake (fat reduced to 18%)
	2. Protein	Extra protein is usually unnecessary during exercise training
	3. Vitamins	More than the RDA of most vitamins is not recommended for the active individual
	4. Antioxidants	Although still controversial, vitamins C and E, beta carotene, zinc and selenium may have beneficial effects in people who exercise regularly.
Food Safety	1. Foodborne infections	Salmonella - due to undercooked chicken, eggs, and meat
	2. Food additives	Nitrites - lengthen storage time but have been implicated in some cancers
	3. Organically grown foods	Grown without the use of pesticides - less toxic but more expensive
	4. Irradiated foods	X-rays used to kill bacteria on foods - data suggest it is a safe practice
	5. Animals treated with drugs	Drugs given to protect animals from disease or increase meat yield - unknown long-term effects on humans

LAB ACTIVITIES

LABORATORY 7.1   (Page 187)

Students should complete the *Diet Analysis* laboratory (Laboratory 7.1). The purpose of this exercise is to analyze eating habits during a 3-day period.

LABORATORY 7.2   (Page 191)

Students should complete the *Construct a New Diet* laboratory (Laboratory 7.2). The purpose of this exercise is to construct a new diet using the principles outlined in Chapter 7.

DISCUSSION ACTIVITIES

- In a class discussion, debate the role of macro- and micro-nutrients in the diet.
- Have the class gather recent news articles about antioxidants and their role in health and exercise.
- Divide the class into groups and have each design a one-day diet choosing foods from the "eating right pyramid" and then discuss the pros and cons of each.

SUGGESTED STUDENT ACTIVITIES

- Have a nutritionist talk to the class about general dietary guidelines.
- Have the class visit a hospital dietitian to learn about special dietary considerations in various disease states.
- Have a sports/exercise nutritionist talk to the class about exercise and nutrition.

SUPPLEMENTAL READINGS

Clark, N. Fluid facts: What, When, and How Much to Drink. Physician and Sports Medicine. 20(11):34-36, 1992.

Connor, S. and W. Connor. New American Diet Systems. New York: Simon and Schuster, 1992.

Fennema, O. The Placebo Effect of Foods. Food Technology. December, 1984, pp. 57-67.

Goodman, M.N., and N.B. Ruderman. Influence of Muscle Use on Amino Acid Metabolism. Exercise and Sports Sciences Reviews. 10: 1-25, 1982.

Hamilton, E., E. Whitney, and F. Sizer. *Nutrition Concepts and Controversies.* St. Paul, MN: West, 1992.

McArdle, W.D., F.I. Katch, and V.L. Katch. Exercise Physiology: Energy, Nutrition, and Human Performance. Lea & Febiger Publishers, Philadelphia, PA, 1991.

Morgan, B.L.G. The Lifelong Nutrition Guide. Prentice-Hall, Englewood Cliffs, NJ, 1983.

Neiman, David C. Fitness and Sports Medicine: An Introduction. Bull Publishing Co., Palo Alto, CA. 1990

Nutrition Action Healthletter. Washington, DC. Center for Science in the Public Interest. 1501 16th St. NW, Washingtion, DC 20036.

EXAM QUESTIONS

MULTIPLE CHOICE
1. The study of food and the way the body uses it to produce energy and build or repair body tissues is defined as:
   a. sports nutrition
   b. nutrition
   c. dietetics
   d. bioenergetics
   Answer: b, page 155, factual

2. Substances contained in food that are necessary for good health are called:
   a. nutrients
   b. by-products
   c. herbs
   d. preservatives
   Answer: a, page 156, factual

3. Which of the following are macronutrients?
   a. vitamins
   b. minerals
   c. protein
   d. antioxidants
   Answer: c, page 156, factual

4. Which of the following are macronutrients?
   a. fats
   b. vitamins
   c. salt
   d. minerals
   Answer: a, page 156, factual

5. The primary function of protein in the diet is to serve as:
   a. a form of energy storage
   b. enzymes for biochemical reactions
   c. building blocks for tissue
   d. nerve chemicals
   Answer: c, page 156, factual

6. The average diet in the U.S. consists of approximately what percentage of fat?
    a. 5
    b. 10
    c. 40
    d. 80
    Answer: c, page 157, factual

7. Which of the following should compose the majority of carbohydrates in a healthy diet?
    a. amino acids
    b. simple carbohydrates
    c. complex carbohydrates
    d. fructose
    Answer: c, page 157, factual

8. Which form of carbohydrate is the only one used by the body in its natural form?
    a. fructose
    b. lactose
    c. maltose
    d. glucose
    Answer: d, page 157, factual

9. The storage form of glucose in muscle and liver cells is called:
    a. galactose
    b. lactose
    c. glycogen
    d. lactic acid
    Answer: c, page 157, factual

10. The stringy, non-digestible carbohydrate found in whole grains, vegetables, and fruits is called:
    a. starch
    b. protein
    c. fructose
    d. fiber
    Answer: d, page 158, factual

11. Cells which store fat are called:
    a. fascia
    b. adipose tissue
    c. cartilage
    d. reticulocytes
    Answer: b, page 159, factual

12. In addition to providing energy, fat also acts to store:
    a. minerals
    b. vitamins
    c. water
    d. electrolytes

Answer: b, page 159, factual

13. Most of the fat stored in the body is classified as:
    a. phospholipids
    b. cholesterol
    c. triglycerides
    d. LDL
    Answer: c, page 159, factual

14. Which of the following comes from animal sources and is solid at room temperature?
    a. vegetable oil
    b. unsaturated fats
    c. saturated fats
    d. starches
    Answer: c, page 159, factual

15. Which of the following is important to the diet but contains no value in providing energy for the body?
    a. sucrose
    b. fatty acids
    c. fiber
    d. fructose
    Answer: c, page 159, conceptual

16. Which of the following is thought to be the major promoter of fatty plaque build-up in the coronary arteries?
    a. unsaturated fats
    b. omega-3 fatty acids
    c. saturated fats
    d. protein
    Answer: c, page 160, factual

17. Which of the following comprise lipoproteins?
    a. protein
    b. triglycerides
    c. cholesterol
    d. all of these
    Answer: d, page 160, factual

18. The best example of the class of fats called derived fats is:
    a. triglycerides
    b. cholesterol
    c. saturated fatty acids
    d. phospholipids
    Answer: b, page 161, factual

19. The basic structural unit of proteins is the:
    a. amino acid

b. polypeptide
c. lipoprotein
d. essential proteins
Answer: a, page 161, factual

20. Micronutrients consist of which of the following?
    a. vitamin B
    b. calcium
    c. iron
    d. all of these
    Answer: d, page 163, factual

21. Which of the following are classified as vitamins?
    a. calcium
    b. magnesium
    c. iron
    d. none of these
    Answer: d, page 163, factual

22. What percentage of the body is water?
    a. 30
    b. 50
    c. 60
    d. 80
    Answer: c, page 168, factual

23. Total daily fat intake should be what percentage of the total caloric intake?
    a. < 30
    b. 30 - 35
    c. 35-40
    d. 40-45
    Answer: a, page 168, factual

24. Of the total fat intake, what percentage should come from saturated fats?
    a. < 10
    b. 15-20
    c. 20-25
    d. none of the above
    Answer: a, page 168, factual

25. Which of the following describes the caloric content of carbohydrate, fat and
    protein, respectively?
    a. 4, 9, 4
    b. 4, 4, 9
    c. 9, 4, 4
    d. none of these
    Answer: a, page 171, factual

26. Nutritional labels on food are based on a diet of _____ calories.

a. 1500
b. 1800
c. 2000
d. 2400
Answer: c, page 173, factual

27. The recommended daily intake of salt is:
    a. < 1000 mg
    b. < 2000 mg
    c. < 2500 mg
    d. < 3000 mg
    Answer: d, page 174, factual

28. A deficiency of iron in the diet would result in:
    a. decreased growth
    b. bone loss
    c. decreased oxygen transport
    d. skin rash
    Answer: c, page 179, factual

29. Which of the following foods should be avoided to maintain a healthy diet?
    a. those high saturated fat
    b. those high in minerals
    c. those high in fiber
    d. those high in vitamins
    Answer: a, page 173, factual

30. Females should be extra cautious to include which of the following in their diet.
    a. iron, calcium
    b. vitamins, phosphorus
    c. potassium, calcium
    d. potassium, sodium
    Answer: a, page 173, factual

31. The increase in calories needed for exercise training should come from which of
    the following macronutrient sources?
    a. fat
    b. protein
    c. carbohydrate
    d. equal portions of each
    Answer: c, page 180, factual

32. Which of the following are recommended to avoid foodborne infections?
    a. wash utensils with soap and hot water after contact with raw poultry
    b. cook all shellfish thoroughly; steaming open may not be sufficient
    c. drink only pasteurized milk
    d. all of the above
    Answer: d, page 183, factual

TRUE / FALSE

33. Nutrition is the study of food and the way the body uses it.
    a. True
    b. False
    Answer: a, page 155, factual

34. Over one-half of all deaths in the United States are associated with health problems linked to poor nutrition.
    a. True
    b. False
    Answer: a, page 155, factual

35. Nutrients are substances contained in foods that are necessary for good health.
    a. True
    b. False
    Answer: a, page 156, factual

36. Carbohydrates, fat and salt are macronutrients necessary for energy transfer in the body.
    a. True
    b. False
    Answer: b, page 156, conceptual

37. A well-balanced diet should consist of approximately 58% carbohydrates, 30% fat, and 12% protein.
    a. True
    b. False
    Answer: a, page 156, factual

38. Fats and carbohydrates serve as the primary fuels to produce energy.
    a. True
    b. False
    Answer: a, page 156, factual

39. The average diet in the U.S. consists of approximately 24% simple sugars.
    a. True
    b. False
    Answer: a, page 157, factual

40. Most carbohydrates in the diet should be composed of simple sugars.
    a. True
     b. False
    Answer: b, page 157, factual

41. Fructose is the only form of carbohydrate which can be used by the body as a fuel.
    a. True
    b. False
    Answer: b, page 157, factual

42. Glycogen is the storage form of glucose in muscle and liver cells.
    a. True
    b. False
    Answer: a, page 157, factual

43. Carbohydrates contain approximately 9 kcal/gram:
    a. True
    b. False
    Answer: b, page 158, factual

44. Both carbohydrate and protein contain approximately 4 kcal/gram.
    a. True
    b. False
    Answer: a, page 158, factual

45. Complex carbohydrates contain both micronutrients and the glucose necessary
    for producing energy.
    a. True
    b. False
    Answer: a, page 158, factual

46. Starch is a long chain of sugars commonly found in foods such as corn, grains,
    potatoes, peas, and beans.
    a. True
    b. False
    Answer: a, page 158, factual

47. Essential fatty acids are those that are necessary in the diet.
    a. True
    b. False
    Answer: a, page 159, factual

48. The most common form of simple fats is cholesterol.
    a. True
    b. False
    Answer: b, page 161, factual

49. Unsaturated fatty acids are those that come from animal sources and are solid at
    room temperature.
    a. True
    b. False
    Answer: b, page 159, factual

50. Fiber is important to the diet but does not contribute to the body's energy needs.
    a. True
    b. False
    Answer: a, page 158, conceptual

51. Omega-3 fatty acids promote fatty plaque build-up in the coronary arteries.

a. True
b. False
Answer: b, page 160, factual

52. Lipoproteins are important because of their role in coronary artery disease.
    a. True
    b. False
    Answer: a, page 160, factual

53. Cholesterol is an example of the class of fats called phospholipids.
    a. True
    b. False
    Answer: b, page 160, factual

54. Amino acid is another name for protein.
    a. True
    b. False
    Answer: b, page 161, factual

55. Micronutrients are necessary for converting food stuffs to useful energy for muscle contraction.
    a. True
    b. False
    Answer: a, page 162, conceptual

56. If not consumed in the diet, micronutrients can be manufactured by the body in times of need.
    a. True
    b. False
    Answer: b, page 163, conceptual

57. The body is approximately 75% water.
    a. True
    b. False
    Answer: b, page 168, factual

58. Saturated fat should constitute < 20% of the total daily caloric intake from fat.
    a. True
    b. False
    Answer: b, page 168, factual

59. Calcium is the most abundant mineral in the body.
    a. True
    b. False
    Answer: a, page 179, factual

60. Athletes need large amounts of protein in the diet to provide energy for training.
    a. True
    b. False

Answer: b, page 168, factual

60. The primary nutritional problem related to simple sugars is that they are not nutrient-dense.
    a. True
    b. False
    Answer: a, page 171, factual

62. The average diet in the U.S. contains 3-10 teaspoons per day of salt.
    a. True
    b. False
    Answer: a, page 174, factual

63. Most U.S. citizens consume half of their dietary intake of carbohydrates in the form of sucrose and corn syrup.
    a. True
    b. False
    Answer: a, page 176, factual

64. Alcohol provides calories to the diet but no micronutrients.
    a. True
    b. False
    Answer: a, page 176, factual

65. Extra protein is needed in the diet of individuals involved in strength training.
    a. True
    b. False
    Answer: b, page 181, factual

66. Some vitamins may be beneficial as antioxidants by protecting cells against free radical damage.
    a. True
    b. False
    Answer: b, page 182, factual

67. The use of radiation to kill microorganisms that grow on food has been shown to be safe and effective.
    a. True
    b. False
    Answer: a, page 183, factual

DISCUSSION

68. What are the macronutrients and why are they important to health?
    Answer: page 156

69. List some common sources of carbohydrates, fats, and proteins in a healthy diet.
    Answer: page 158

70. Compare simple and complex carbohydrates and tell the importance of each.
    Answer: page 158

71. Discuss the various types of fats and how they are used by the body.
    Answer: page 159

72. Discuss the role of water in the diet.
    Answer: page 168

73. What is the importance of vitamins in the diet and are supplements necessary?
    Answer: page 163

74. What is the role of minerals in the body?
    Answer: page 163

75. In order to have a healthy diet, what types of foods should be removed from the diet of most individuals.
    Answer: page 172

76. Discuss the special dietary mineral requirements for females.
    Answer: page 179

77. Discuss the special nutrient needs for an individual participating in a physical fitness program.
    Answer: page 180

Chapter 8
Exercise, Diet, and Weight Control

CHAPTER SUMMARY

1. Millions of people in the U.S. are carrying too much body fat for optimal health.

2. Obesity is defined as a high percentage of body fat; over 25% for men and over 30% for women.

3. Obesity is linked to many diseases including heart disease, diabetes, and hypertension.

4. The optimal percent body fat for health and fitness is believed to be 10-20% (men) and 15-25% (women).

5. The energy balance theory of weight control states that to maintain your body weight, your energy intake must equal your energy expenditure.

6. Evidence suggests that creating a fat deficit is an essential factor in weight loss. This is because dietary fat is more easily stored as body fat than either carbohydrate or protein. The importance of a low fat diet in weight control is illustrated by the fact that body fat gain is a result of a continual imbalance of fat intake and fat metabolism .

7. Total daily energy expenditure is the sum of both resting metabolic rate and exercise metabolic rate.

8. The four basic components of a comprehensive weight control program are: 1) weight loss goals; 2) a reduced caloric diet stressing balanced nutrition; 3) a exercise program designed to increase caloric expenditure and maintain muscle mass; and 4) a behavior modification program designed to modify those behaviors that contribute to weight gain.

9. Weight loss goals should include both short-term and long-term goals.

10. Numerous weight loss myths exist. This chapter has discredited diet pills, spot reduction, grapefruit diets, cellulite reduction, and the use of saunas, steam baths, and rubber suits to promote weight loss.

11. Two relatively common eating disorders are anorexia nervosa and bulimia. Both are serious medical problems and require professional treatment.

12. Weight training and a positive caloric balance are both required to produce increases in muscle mass.

LEARNING OBJECTIVES

After reading this chapter you should be able to do the following:

1. Define obesity and discuss potential causes of obesity.

2. From a disease perspective, explain why obesity is considered to be unhealthy.

3. Explain the concept of optimal body weight.

4. Discuss the energy balance theory of weight control.

5. Explain the roles of resting metabolic rate and exercise metabolic rate in determining daily energy expenditure.

6. Outline a simple method to estimate your daily caloric expenditure.

7. List and define the four basic components of a weight loss program.

8. Discuss several weight loss myths.

9. Define the eating disorders anorexia nervosa and bulimia.

10. Discuss strategies to gain body weight.

LECTURE OUTLINE

Key Points	Subpoints	Examples
Obesity refers to a high percentage of body	1. Sixty-five million people in the U.S. are obese	obesity is defined as: males >25% fat females > 30% fat

Key Points	Subpoints	Examples
Obesity is a health risk	1. Obesity increases the risk for 26 different diseases	Heart disease, colon cancer, hypertension, type II diabetes, etc.
There is no single cause of obesity genetics and life style	1. Obesity is related to both	Children of obese parents have a greater risk of becoming obese
Regional fat storage	1. Site for body fat storage is genetically determined	
Optimal body fat	1. Researchers disagree on exact percentages of body fat that is considered optimal	Optimal % body fat Males = 10-20% Females = 15-25%
Energy balance concept of weight control	1. To maintain a constant body weight, your energy intake must equal your energy expenditure	Isocaloric diet = (energy intake = energy expenditure)
Energy expenditure	1. Total daily energy expenditure = resting metabolic rate + exercise metabolic rate	Techniques exist to estimate daily caloric expenditure
Fat deficit concept of weight control	1. Creating a fat deficit is essential in fat loss	Fat deficit = fat usage > fat intake
What is a safe rate of weight loss?	1. One pound per week is generally considered safe	3500 Kcal/pound of fat Therefore, caloric deficit of 500 Kcal/day would result in a fat loss of one pound/day

Key Points	Subpoints	Examples
Establishing a successful weight loss program	Four basic components of a comprehensive weight loss program include: 1. Establishing weight loss goals 2. Reduced caloric diet that stresses balanced nutrition 3. Exercise program 4. Behavior modification program aimed at changing eating behavior	
Key points associated with a safe diet	1. Low in calories but contains essential nutrients 2. Low in fat 3. Diet should contain a variety of foods 4. Diet should be compatible with lifestyle 5. Diet should be lifelong 6. Diet should contain healthy foods	< 30% total calories in fat Foods easily obtained That is, a diet that can be followed throughout life
Exercise and weight loss	1. Exercise plays a key role in weight loss	Both low and high intensity exercise can assist in weight loss programs
Behavior modification is a key factor in achieving both short-term and long-term weight loss	1. Eating behaviors are learned and behavior modification is a means of eliminating improper eating habits	Social or environmental stimuli often promote eating behaviors (i.e. eating popcorn at movies)

79

Key Points	Subpoints	Examples
Weight loss myths	1. Diet pills	Over-the-counter diet pills often
	2. Spot reduction	contain caffeine and have not been
	3. Grapefruit diet	shown to be effective in long-term
	4. Eating before bed	weight loss
	5. Cellulite	Cellulite is lumpy fat
	6. Fat dissolving creams	Fat dissolving creams are not
		effective
	7. Saunas, steam baths, and rubber suits	Heat does not dissolve fat
Eating disorders include:	1. The incidence of eating disorders has grown in recent years	Two common eating disorders 1. Anorexia Nervosa 2. Bulimia
Exercise and diet programs to gain weight	1. Body weight gain can be achieved in two ways: a) Increase body fat b) Increase lean body mass (e.g. muscle mass)	Create positive caloric balance Engage in resistance training

LAB ACTIVITIES
LABORATORY 8.1, page 217
LABORATORY 8.2, page 219
LABORATORY 8.3, page 221

This chapter provides three laboratory exercises. *Laboratory 8-1* provides an opportunity for students to compute their ideal body weight using both percent body fat and the body mass index. *Laboratory 8-2* permits the estimation of daily caloric expenditure and the caloric deficit required to lose one pound of body fat. Finally, *Laboratory 8-3* is a log book to record weight loss goals and progress.

DISCUSSION ACTIVITIES
• Organize discussion groups to discuss the concept of optimal body weight.

• Have a class discussion concerning the importance of exercise and behavior modification in achieving weight loss goals.

• Invite a local obesity and/or weight loss expert to discuss some aspect of weight loss.

SUGGESTED STUDENT ACTIVITIES

• Visit a local eating disorder clinic and have an expert on this topic discuss the importance of recognizing the symptoms and treating eating disorders.

SUPPLEMENTAL READINGS

American College of Sports Medicine. (L. Durstine et al. Eds.)Resource Manual for Guidelines for Exercise Testing and Prescription, Second Edition. Lea and Febiger, Philadelphia. 1993.

Getchell, B. Physical Fitness: A Way of Life. Macmillan Publishing Company, New York. 1992.

Powers, S. and E. Howley. Exercise Physiology: Theory and Application to Fitness and Performance. Brown and Benchmark, Dubuque, IA, 1994.

Williams, M. Lifetime Fitness and Wellness. Brown and Benchmark, Dubuque, IA. 1996.

EXAM QUESTIONS

Multiple choice

1. Obesity is defined as
   a. a large percent of body fat
   b. >25% fat in men
   c. >30% fat in women
   d. all of above are correct
   answer: d, factual, page 195

2. Obesity is linked to an increased risk of
   a. heart disease
   b. brain cancer
   c. dementia
   d. none of above are correct
   answer: a, factual, page 196

81

3. The optimal percent body fat for men is estimated to be
   a. 5-10%
   b. 10-20%
   c. 15-25%
   d. >25%
   answer: b, factual, page 198

4. The optimal percent body fat for women is estimated to be
   a. 10-15%
   b. 10-20%
   c. 15-25%
   d. 20-35%
   answer: c, factual, page 198

5. Total daily caloric expenditure is defined as
   a. the sum of resting and basal metabolic rate
   b. the sum of basal and exercise metabolic rate
   c. the sum of resting and exercise metabolic rate
   d. none of above
   answer: c, factual, page 199-200

6. Which of the following is not a component of a comprehensive weight loss program?
   a. weight loss goals
   b. reduced caloric intake
   c. exercise program
   d. yoga program
   answer: d, factual, page 199-203

7. It is believed that _____% of adult women in the U.S. are on a diet.
   a. 10
   b. 20-25
   c. 30-40
   d. 60-70
   answer: c, factual, page 195

8. Obesity increases the risk of at least _____ diseases

a. 5

b. 10

c. 20

d. 26

answer: d, factual, page 196

9. Consuming more calories that you expend is termed

    a. a negative caloric balance

    b. a positive caloric balance

    c. an isocaloric balance

    d. none of above are correct

    answer: b, factual, page 199

10. The maximum rate of weight loss is approximately _____ pounds per week.

    a. 1-2

    b. 3-4

    c. 4-5

    d. 6-10

    answer: a, factual, page 201-202

11. The primary factor that determines where (body location) body fat is stored is

    a) the type of food eaten

    b. the somatotype

    c. genetics

    d. none of above are correct

    answer: c, factual, page 197

12. A positive caloric balance is defined as

    a. food intake equals energy expenditure

    b. consuming more calories than expended

    c. expending more calories than consumed

    d. none of above are correct

    answer: b, factual, page 199

13. The maximal safe rate of weight loss is _____ pounds per week.

    a. 1-2

b. 3-5

c. 6-8

d. 9-10

answer: a, factual, page 201

14. Which of the following statements concerning diet are true?

a. the diet should be low in fat (e.g. <30% total calories)

b. the diet should employ a variety of foods to provide total nutrition

c. the diet should be low in calories but high in nutrients

d. all of above are true

answer: d, factual, page 203

15. Moderate exercise has been shown to

a. increase appetite by 70%

b. increase appetite by 45%

c. decrease appetite by -40%

d. have little influence on appetite

answer: d, factual, page 206

True/False

16. It is well established that diet pills provide a safe and productive means of losing body fat.

a. true

b. false

answer: b, factual, page 208

17. Evidence suggests that creating a fat deficit is essential in losing body fat.

a. true

b. false

answer: a, factual, page 201

18. Dietary fat is more easily stored as body fat compared to dietary carbohydrate or protein.

a. true

b. false

answer: a, factual, page 201

19. Weight loss goals should only focus on "short-term goals".
   a. true
   b. false
   answer: b, factual, page 203-204

20. Exercise does not play a key role in weight loss.
   a. true
   b. false
   answer: b, factual, page 204

21. Most diet experts recommend a weight loss diet that is nutritionally balanced.
   a. true
   b. false
   answer: a, factual, page 203

22. It is well established that moderate exercise training results in a large increase in appetite.
   a. true
   b. false
   answer: b, factual, page 206

23. Eating highly acidic grapefruit has been shown to reduce body fat.
   a. true
   b. false
   answer: b, factual, page 208

24. An intense fear of gaining weight may be a symptom of anorexia nervosa.
   a. true
   b. false
   answer: a, factual, page 210

25. Weight training and a positive caloric balance will result in an increase in muscle mass.
   a. true

b. false

answer: a, factual, page 211-212

26. Obesity is a term applied to people with a high percentage of body fat.

    a. true

    b. false

    answer: a, factual, page 195

27. The additional gain of body fat slowly over a period of years is commonly called "creeping obesity".

    a. true

    b. false

answer: a, factual, page 196

28. Men tend to store body fat in the lower body whereas many women store body fat in the upper body.

    a. true

    b. false

    answer: b, factual, page 197

29. An isocaloric balance is defined as consuming more calories than the body expends during the day.

    a. true

    b. false

    answer: b, factual, page 199

30. The set point theory of weight control centers around the concept that body weight is controlled at a set point by a weight-regulating control center within the brain.

    a. true

    b. false

    answer: a, factual, page 199

31. Resting metabolic rate is the amount of energy expended during sleep.

    a. true

    b. false

    answer: a, factual, page 200

32. The maximal recommended rate of weight loss is 4-5 pounds per week.
    a. true
    b. false
    answer: b, factual, page 201

32. When losing body fat, most of the fat loss occurs in body areas that contain the most fat.
    a. true
    b. false
    answer: a, factual, page 202

33. The establishment of weight loss goals is not a key component to a weight loss program.
    a. true
    b. false
    answer: b, factual, page 203

34. A balanced diet should contain fruits, vegetables, and whole grains.
    a. true
    b. false
    answer: a, factual, page 203

35. Regular aerobic exercise results in an improved ability to burn fat as energy.
    a. true
    b. false
    answer: b,conceptual, page 204

36. An exercise program designed to assist in weight loss should contain only cardiorespiratory training.
    a. true
    b. false
    answer: b, factual, page 204

37. Behavior modification is a technique used in psychological therapy to promote desirable changes in behavior.

a. true

b. false

answer: a, factual, page 206

38. The performance of "sit-ups" will result in spot reduction of body fat.

a. true

b. false

answer: b, factual, page 208

39. Eating highly acidic foods like grapefruit will dissolve fat.

a. true

b. false

answer: b, factual, page 208

40. A common symptom of anorexia nervosa is a fear of gaining weight.

a. true

b. false

answer: a, factual, page 210

Discussion

41. What is obesity? What diseases are linked to obesity? page 196

42. Discuss several possible causes of obesity. page 196

43. Discuss the concept of optimal body weight. How is the optimal body weight computed? pages 197-198

44. Explain the roles of resting metabolic rate (RMR) and exercise metabolic rate (EMR) in determining total caloric expenditure. Which is more important in total daily caloric expenditure in a sedentary individual? pages 200-201

45. Outline a simple method that can be used to compute your daily caloric expenditure. Give an example. page 200-201

46. List the four major components of a weight loss program. page 203

47. Discuss the following weight loss myths: 1) spot reduction; 2) grapefruit diet; 3) eating before bed; 4) cellulite; and 5) saunas, steam baths, and rubber suits. page 208-209

48. Define the eating disorders, anorexia nervosa and bulimia. pages 210

49. Discuss the role of behavior modification in weight loss. pages 206-207

50. Define the following terms:

> energy balance theory of weight control
>
> isocaloric balance
>
> negative caloric balance
>
> positive caloric balance
>
> set point theory
>
> page 199

51. Explain the fat deficit concept of weight control. page 201

52. Compare exercise metabolic rate and resting metabolic rate. page 200

53. What is cellulite? page 208-209

54. How does creeping obesity occur? pages 196-197

55. Discuss the process of combining diet and exercise to increase muscle mass. pages 211-212

89

Chapter 9
Exercise and the Environment

CHAPTER SUMMARY

1. Evaporation is the primary means of heat loss during exercise in a hot environment.

2. While it is generally safe to exercise in a hot environment, the following guidelines need consideration:

   a) start slow and reduce your total exercise time.

   b) Adjust your exercise intensity to avoid exceeding your target heart rate.

   c) Wear loose, light colored clothing.

   d) Drink plenty of fluids before, during, and after the exercise session.

3. Heat acclimatization occurs after several days of exposure to a hot environment. It results in a greater ability to loose body heat and reduces the chance of heat injury.

4. Although long-term exercise in a cold environment could result in hypothermia, in general, short-term exercise in a cold environment does not pose a serious threat to heat balance.

5. Exercise at high altitude results in a reduced amount of oxygen in the arterial blood which reduces oxygen transport to the working muscles and lowers both VO_2 max and exercise tolerance.

6. At altitude, it is necessary to reduce the intensity of exercise below normal in order to stay within your target heart rate range. However, there is little need to reduce your duration or frequency of exercise training during brief stays at moderate altitudes.

7. Ozone is produced by a chemical reaction between sunlight and automobile exhaust. Carbon monoxide is produced by the burning of fossil fuels. Both forms of air pollution can impair exercise tolerance.

8. The best way to deal with air pollution is to avoid exercising when ozone or carbon monoxide levels are high. Ozone levels are highest during hot summer days. Carbon monoxide levels are highest when automobile traffic is heavy.

LEARNING OBJECTIVES

After studying this chapter, the student should be able to:

1. Describe how to prevent heat loss during exercise.
2. List several important guidelines for exercising in a hot environment.
3. Describe the appropriate exercise clothing for exercising in the heat.
4. Differentiate between the various types of heat injuries.
5. Discuss how heat acclimatization reduces the risk of heat injury.
6. Describe the appropriate clothing for exercise in a cold environment.
7. Explain why exercise at high altitude results in higher heart rate and elevated breathing.
8. List two major forms of air pollution.
9. Outline a strategy for coping with air pollution.

LECTURE OUTLINE

Key Points	Subpoints	Examples
Problems with exercise	1. Maximizing heat loss is essential in the heat	Primary means - convection and evaporation (high humidity retards evaporation)
	2. Guidelines for exercising in the heat	Note the dangers of high temperature and humidity (see Figure 9.3)
		Use "target heart rate" (Chapter 4) as a guide to intensity when exercising in the heat
	3. Optimizing clothing when exercising in the heat	Minimize clothing - it should be light-colored, lightweight, and allow air to pass
	4. Lack of heat acclimation	Retarded sweat rate, less evaporative cooling, loss of blood volume
		10-12 days needed for heat acclimation
		Higher incidence of heat injuries - heat cramps, heat exhaustion, and heatstroke

Key Points	Subpoints	Examples
Problems with exercise	1. Maintaining body temperature in the cold is essential	A combination of heat production and body insulation is necessary to maintain body temperature.
	2. Proper clothing is critical	Optimal clothing should - be layered to trap air for best insulation, prevent sweating, permit sweat loss, should it occur, to the atmosphere.
	3. Wind decreases the "effective" temperature	Understand the "wind-chill factor" and use extra precautions (see Figure 9.5)
Problems with exercise	1. Primary problem is decreased oxygen delivery to muscle	Decreased VO2 max and exercise capacity at altitude
	2. Physiological adjustments must take place	Increased heart rate and breathing
Problems with exercise in polluted air	1. Air pollution irritates lungs and decreases oxygen delivery to muscles	Ozone and carbon monoxide are primary pollutants
	2. Guidelines to combat air pollution	Try to avoid exercise when ozone and carbon monoxide levels are high (see Figure 9.8) Avoid exercise in high traffic areas

LAB ACTIVITIES

No laboratories are included in this chapter

DISCUSSION ACTIVITIES

- If any students have been to extremely high altitude, have them tell the class about the experience.
- If any students have been in extremely hot or cold environments, have them tell the class about the experience.
- Discuss the importance of fluid replacement during exercise in the heat.
- Discuss the role of electrolyte replacement during exercise in the heat.

SUGGESTED STUDENT ACTIVITIES

• Have students contact the local health department to determine the levels of air pollution in the community.

• Have students visit a local meteorologist to learn how the "heat index" and "wind-chill factor" are determined.

SUPPLEMENTAL READINGS

Fox, E., R. Bowers, and M. Foss. The Physiological Basis for Exercise and Sport. Brown & Benchmark Publishers, Dubuque, Iowa, 1993.

Neiman, David C. Fitness and Sports Medicine: An Introduction. Bull Publishing Co., Palo Alto, CA. 1990

Powers, S.K. and E. T. Howley. Exercise Physiology: Theory and Application to Fitness and Performance. Brown & Benchmark Publishers, Dubuque, Iowa, 1994.

West, J.B. and S. Lahiri, eds. High Altitude and Man. Williams & Wilkins, Inc., Baltimore, MD, 1984.

EXAM QUESTIONS

MULTIPLE CHOICE

1. Humans regulate their body temperature around:
    a. 97° F (35° C)
    b. 98.6° F (37° C)
    c. 99° F (39° C)
    d. 93° F (33° C)
    Answer: b, page 225, factual

2. Which of the following would be an indication of impending heat illness?
    a. nausea
    b. profuse sweating
    c. cold, clammy skin
    d. hunger
    Answer: a, page 225, factual

3. Which of the following is a major mechanism of heat loss during exercise?
    a. conduction
    b. radiation
    c. evaporation
    d. diffusion
    Answer: c, page 226, factual

4. At a given metabolic rate and heat production, which of the following exercises would allow the most cooling through convection?
    a. running
    b. walking

c. cycling
d. lifting weights
Answer: a, page 225, conceptual

5. During exercise, body temperature would rise to the highest level in which of the following environmental conditions?
   a. high temperature / low humidity
   b. high temperature / high humidity
   c. low temperature / high humidity
   c. low temperature / low humidity
   Answer: b, page 226, conceptual

6. The best way to determine if the environmental conditions are imposing a heat load on your body during exercise is to monitor your:
   a. breathing
   b. sweat rate
   c. heart rate
   d. skin temperature
   Answer: c, page 228, factual

7. Which of the following would best describe clothing which should be worn during exercise in the heat.
   a. lightweight
   b. allows air to pass through
   c. light in color
   d. all of the above
   Answer: d, page 229, conceptual

8. The physiological adaptations that occur to assist the body in dissipating heat is called:
   a. growth
   b. habituation
   c. acclimatization
   d. homeostasis
   Answer: c, page 230, factual

9. Which of the following is an adaptation that the body makes to chronic heat stress?
   a. lower sweat rate
   b. reduced glucose in the blood
   c. lower blood volume
   d. earlier onset of sweating
   Answer: d, page 230, factual

10. Acclimatization to heat stress occurs in approximately:
    a. 3-4 days
    b. 10-12 days
    c. 16-20 days
    d. > 3 weeks
    Answer: b, page 230, factual

11. Which of the following is characterized by muscle spasms and twitching of limbs?
   a. heat cramps
   b. heat exhaustion
   c. heat stroke
   d. none of the above
   Answer: a, page 230, factual

12. Which of the following is characterized by weakness, fatigue, decreased blood pressure, blurred vision, and pale, clammy skin.
   a. heat cramps
   b. heat exhaustion
   c. heat stroke
   d. none of the above
   Answer: b, page 230, factual

13. Which of the following is characterized by lack of sweating, limp muscles, seizures and vomiting.
   a. heat cramps
   b. heat exhaustion
   c. heat stroke
   d. none of the above
   Answer: c, page 230, factual

14. Which of the following are common to all heat illness conditions?
   a. initiated by exercise
   b. significant loss of water
   c. increased heat storage by the body
   d. all of the above
   Answer: d, page 232, factual

15. Some combination of heat production and warm clothing are necessary to maintain body temperature at ambient temperatures of less than:
   a. 80° F
   b. 60° F
   c. 40° F
   d. 32° F
   Answer: b, page 232, factual

16. The best strategy for dressing to exercise in the cold is:
   a. wear the thickest garment available
   b. wear light colored clothes
   c. wear clothing which retards moisture penetration
   d. wear layers of clothing
   Answer: d, page 232, conceptual

17. The phenomenon of wind movement causing a loss of body heat is caused by:
   a. conduction
   b. radiation

b. False

Answer: b, page 232, factual

34. The wind-chill factor refers to the fact that exposure of skin to a cold environment can cause skin to freeze.
    a. True
    b. False

    Answer: b, page 233, factual

35. The primary concern with exercise at altitude is the fact that there is less oxygen in the air.
    a. True
    b. False

    Answer: b, page 233, factual

36. The greater the altitude, the greater the reduction in VO_2 max.
    a. True
    b. False

    Answer: a, page 233, factual

37. The primary forms of air pollution that affect exercise performance are ozone and nitrogen.
    a. True
    b. False

    Answer: b, page 235, factual

38. Carbon monoxide causes a decrease in oxygen transport to muscles during exercise.
    a. True
    b. False

    Answer: a, page 234, factual

39. To avoid exercising when ozone is high, it is best to avoid exercise between 5-6 in the evening.
    a. True
    b. False

    Answer: b, page 235, factual

40. Since air pollution is visible, it is easy to determine when not to exercise.
    a. True
    b. False

    Answer: b, page 235, factual

DISCUSSION

41. Discuss the mechanisms of heat loss during exercise.
    Answer: page 226

42. Discuss the guidelines for safe exercise in the heat
    Answer: page 228

43. What are the physiological adaptations to chronic heat exposure.
    Answer: page 230

45. What is the best strategy for dressing for exercising in extreme cold?
    Answer: page 232

46. What is the wind-chill factor and what does it mean for exercise in the cold?
    Answer: page 233

46. What physiological alterations occur to help cope with the stress of altitude?
    Answer: page 233

47. What are the major air pollutants which affect exercise performance?
    Answer: page 235

48. Discuss the strategies for exercise training in areas of high air pollution.
    Answer: page 235

Chapter 10
Exercise for Special Populations

CHAPTER SUMMARY

1. Individuals with orthopedic problems often require special considerations when designing an exercise program. The objective of the exercise prescription is to find an exercise mode that increases physical fitness but does not aggravate the existing orthopedic condition.

2. The obese individual should emphasize the use of non-weight-bearing activities (swimming, cycling, etc.). In addition, the exercise should be of lower than normal intensity.

3. Diabetes results from a deficiency in the amount or effectiveness of the hormone insulin which acts to transfer glucose from the blood into the cells.

4. The key to developing a sound exercise program for a type I diabetic is to learn to manage blood glucose levels during exercise. If blood glucose can be managed, the diabetic individual can participate in the same activities as the non-diabetic individual.

5. Only minor differences exist in the exercise guidelines for the type I and the type II diabetic. The most important difference is the recommended duration of exercise (type II diabetics generally perform a longer duration of exercise).

6. Asthma is a disease that results in a sudden reduction in the size of the airways. Asthmatics who can medically control their asthma can safely participate in an exercise training program.

7. Aging is not a sudden process but is a slow, gradual decline in biological function. The common functional changes seen with both aging and inactivity are decreased cardiorespiratory function, obesity, and musculoskeletal fragility. Approximately one-half of the decline in functional capacity observed with aging is due to a decrease in physical activity.

8. Pregnancy does not prevent women from exercising. Short-duration, low-to-moderate intensity exercise does not pose a serious risk to the health of the fetus or the mother.

LEARNING OBJECTIVES

After studying this chapter you should be able to:

1. Describe factors to consider in developing an exercise program for an individual with orthopedic problems.

2. Outline the exercise guidelines for an obese individual.

3. Discuss exercise training programs for type I and type II diabetics.

4. Discuss the benefits of exercise for asthmatics.

5. Outline the considerations for beginning or continuing an exercise program during pregnancy.

6. Discuss the physiological changes seen with aging and list the general guidelines for maintaining an exercise program throughout life.

LECTURE OUTLINE

Key Points	Subpoints	Examples
Benefits of exercise for individuals with special concerns	1. Increased stamina 2. Enhanced quality of life	
Orthopedic problems	1. Use muscle groups distant from injury	For knee pain associated with jogging, substitute swimming
Exercise and obesity	1. Exercise limitations	Heat intolerance, shortness of breath, lack of flexibility, frequent injuries, lack of balance
	2. Emphasize duration	> 30 min. per session with emphasis on energy expenditure-not aerobic fitness Expenditure should be >300 kcal per workout

Key Points	Subpoints	Examples
Exercise and diabetes	1. Define	Types I and II
	2. Management	Diet, exercise and insulin
	3. Exercise benefits	Controls blood glucose
		Controls body weight
		Lowers risk of coronary heart disease
		Psychosocial benefits
	4. Exercise and type I	Normal prescription but performed daily
		Follow safety precautions from physician
	5. Exercise and type II	Emphasis on controlling body weight increase duration and frequency (60 min - 5 days per week)
Exercise and asthma	1. Define	
	2. Safety concerns with exercise	Never exercise alone, carry inhaler, avoid polluted or cold air
Exercise and pregnancy	1. Safety concerns	Avoid - contact sports, lying on your back more than 5 min., exercise where balance is important, heat, weight-bearing exercise.
	2. Exercise prescription	Short-duration, low to moderate intensity
Exercise and aging	1. Physiological changes	Decreased VO2 max and exercise capacity, increased body fat, and musculoskeletal fragility.
	2. Safety concerns	Avoid exercise which creates orthopedic stress such as jogging, get physician clearance before exercising, use non- weight-bearing exercises

Key Points	Subpoints	Examples
	3. Exercise guidelines	Use the lower end of target heart rate range, limit frequency to 3-4 days/week.

LAB ACTIVITIES

No laboratories are included in this chapter

DISCUSSION ACTIVITIES

- Discuss orthopedics problems experienced by students and explore ways to circumvent those with various types of exercise.

- Discuss the safety concerns of exercise for obese individuals. How should the exercise prescription allow for these concerns?

- Ask any students with diabetes to volunteer stories about their management of blood glucose and the role of exercise.

- Discuss how management of asthma can allow normal participation in exercise programs.

- Discuss the potential problems of exercise during pregnancy. What strategies can be employed to allow safe exercise during pregnancy?

SUGGESTED STUDENT ACTIVITIES

- Have an athletic trainer speak to the class on ways to modify the exercise prescription for individuals with various orthopedic injuries.

- If there are students in the class with diabetes, ask them to share their experiences with exercise and the management of blood glucose.

- If there are students in the class with asthma, ask them to share their experiences with breathing during exercise.

SUPPLEMENTAL READINGS

American College of Sports Medicine. Position Statement on Proper and Improper Weight Loss Programs. Medicine and Science in Sports and Exercise. 17:1984.

Artal, R., and R.A. Wiswell. 1986. Exercise in Pregnancy. Williams & Wilkins, Los Angeles, CA

Botti, J.J., and R.L. Jones. Aerobic Conditioning, Nutrition, and Pregnancy. Clinical Nutrition. 4:14-17, 1985.

Bouchard, C., L. Perusse, and C. Leblanc. Inheritance of the Amount and Distribution of Human Body Fat. International Journal of Obesity. 12:205-215. 1988.

Kulpa, P.J., B.M. White, and R. Visscher. Aerobic Exercise in Pregnancy. American Journal of Obstetrics and Gynecology. 156: 1395-1403, 1987.

Larson, E.B. and R.A. Bruce. Health Benefits of Exercise in an Aging Society. Archives of Internal Medicine. 147:353-356, 1987.

Morton, M.J., M.S. Paul, and J. Metcalfe. Exercise During Pregnancy. Medical Clinics of North America. 69:97-107, 1985.

Neiman, David C. 1990 . Fitness and Sports Medicine: An Introduction. Bull Publishing Co., Palo Alto, CA

Powers, S.K. and E. T. Howley. 1994. Exercise Physiology: Theory and Application to Fitness and Performance. Brown & Benchmark Publishers, Dubuque, Iowa

Roberts, J.A. Exercise-induced Asthma in Athletes. Sports Medicine. 6:193-196, 1988.

Stamford, B. A. Exercise and the Elderly. Exercise and Sports Sciences Reviews. 16:341-379, 1988.

EXAM QUESTIONS

MULTIPLE CHOICE

1. Exercise programs for people with orthopedic problems should be designed to:

    a. minimize exercise intensity

    b. maximize the weight used to strengthen muscles

    c. emphasize the use of muscle groups distant to the injury

d. all of the above

Answer: c, page 240, conceptual

2. For an individual with an orthopedic problem, developing aerobic fitness should utilize which of the following:

a. cycling

b. walking

c. swimming

d. all of the above

Answer: a, page 240, conceptual

3. Which of the following would be considered special considerations for exercise in the obese individual?

a. heat intolerance

b. loose joints

c. excess lung capacity

d. all of the above

Answer: a, page 240, factual

4. The primary goal of an exercise program should be to:

a. improve flexibility

b. improve aerobic endurance

c. increase energy expenditure

d. increase lung function

Answer: c, page 240, conceptual

5. Which of the following would be considered appropriate exercise for the obese individual?

a. jogging

b. weight lifting

c. tennis

d. swimming

Answer: d, page 240, conceptual

6. A metabolic disorder characterized by high blood glucose levels is known as:

   a. asthma

   b. scoliosis

   c. diabetes

   d. myasthenia gravis

   Answer: c, page 241, factual

7. Which of the following are important in managing diabetes?

   a. exercise

   b. diet

   c. insulin

   d. all of the above

   Answer: d, page 241, factual

8. With proper diet and exercise, it is estimated that approximately _____ % of non-insulin dependent diabetes could be prevented.

   a. 40

   b. 55

   c. 75

   d. 90

   Answer: d, page 241, factual

9. Which of the following are considered benefits of exercise for the diabetic?

   a. control blood glucose

   b. increases insulin secretion

   c. increases fat metabolism

   d. all of the above

   Answer: a, page 241, conceptual

10. The major objective of exercise for the type II diabetic is to:

a. increase insulin secretion

b. increase carbohydrate metabolism

c. reduce body fat

d. all of the above

Answer: d, page 242, conceptual

11. Which of the following is considered one of the guidelines for exercise training for asthmatics?

a. Participate only in swimming exercise

b. never use your inhaler during exercise

c. never exercise alone

d. try to exercise in cold weather

Answer: d, page 243, conceptual

12. Which of the following is considered one of the guidelines for exercise during pregnancy?

a. exercise on your back when possible

b. exercise in the heat when possible

c. use weight-bearing exercises

d. drink fluids while exercising

Answer: d, page 243, conceptual

13. The primary concern with exercise during pregnancy is the possibility of:

a. reduced blood flow to the fetus

b. heat build-up affecting fetus

c. both of these

d. none of these

Answer: c, page 243, conceptual

14. Which of the following changes occur with age and affect exercise capacity?

a. VO2 max

b. body composition

25. Type II diabetes occurs primarily in adults and is usually non-insulin-dependent.
   a. True
   b. False
   Answer: b, page 241, factual

26. Exercise for the individual with asthma should be performed in cold weather when possible.
   a. True
   b. False
   Answer: b, page 243, factual

27. One of the primary concerns with exercise during pregnancy is that blood flow to the fetus may be compromised during intense exercise.
   a. True
   b. False
   Answer: a, page 243, conceptual

28. Exercise during pregnancy should emphasize activities that require balance and are weight-bearing.
   a. True
   b. False
   Answer: b, page 243, conceptual

29. The VO2 max decreases with age due to biological adaptations which cannot be altered with exercise.
   a. True
   b. False
   Answer: b, page 244, conceptual

30. Exercise frequency should be higher than normal for older individuals.
   a. True
   b. False

Answer: b, page 245, factual

DISCUSSION

31. What is the goal of designing a fitness program for an individual with an orthopedic problem?

    Answer: page 240

32. Discuss the primary purpose of an exercise program for obese individuals.

    Answer: page 240

33. List the types of exercise appropriate for obese individuals and give examples of each.

    Answer: page 241

34. What is the role of exercise in each of the types of diabetes (i.e., types I and II)?

    Answer: page 241

35. How does asthma affect the exercise prescription?

    Answer: page 241

36. Discuss the guidelines for exercise during pregnancy.

    Answer: page 243

37. Discuss the guidelines for exercise for the older individual.

    Answer: page 244

111

Chapter 11
Prevention and Rehabilitation of Exercise-Related Injuries

CHAPTER SUMMARY

1. Injuries involved with running occur primarily in the foot and knee. This is due to the excessive stress placed on the legs and feet. The factors most closely associated with running injuries are improper training techniques, poor equipment, and alignment problems in the legs and feet.

2. Factors associated with injuries in aerobic dance are the number of sessions per week, improper shoes, and non-resilient surfaces.

3. Over-training is the greatest risk to developing an exercise-related injury.

4. Back pain is a multifactoral problem which usually subsides without any medical intervention. Exercise, however, can play an important role in preventing back pain and rehabilitation of some back problems. Exercises to increase flexibility and strength, reduce body fat, improve muscle balance between the trunk flexors and extensors, and prevent osteoporosis can decrease your risk of developing back problems.

5. Acute muscle soreness occurs during or immediately after an exercise bout. This type of injury may be due to muscle damage, accumulation of fluid within the muscle, and/or chemical imbalances within the muscle itself.

6. Delayed-onset muscle soreness (DOMS) usually occurs 24-48 hours after a bout of exercise (eccentric exercise increases the chance DOMS).

7. When muscle is forced to contract against excessive resistance, fibers are damaged. This damage is referred to as a *strain* and can range from a minor separation of fibers to a complete tear.

8. Tendonitis is one of the most common of all overuse problems associated with physical activity. The term literally means inflammation of a tendon.

9. A sprain is caused by damage to a ligament; connective tissue that provides support for joints. In contrast, torn cartilage refers to damage to the tough, connective tissue which serves as a pad between the ends of bones.

10. Common injuries to the lower extremities are: 1) PFPS, in which the articular cartilage on the back of the knee cap (patella) may be damaged by chronic use during exercise, 2) shin splints, which encompasses several different injuries to the front of the lower leg, and 3) stress fractures which are microscopic breaks in the bone.

11. The following steps reduce your risk of developing an exercise-related injury:

   1) Engage in a program of muscle strengthening exercises to keep a balance in strength around joints.

   2) Warm-up before and cool-down after each workout.

   3) Use the proper equipment (including proper footwear).

   4) Increase your exercise intensity and duration slowly throughout your exercise training program.

   5) Maintain the proper rest to exercise ratio. Do not over-train!

12. For treating injuries, remember the R.I.C.E. principle: rest, ice, compression and elevation.

13. Recently, an effective new technique for injury rehabilitation called cryokinetics has come into use. This treatment calls for alternating cold applications and exercise.

LEARNING OBJECTIVES

After studying this chapter, you should be able to:

1) Discuss the role of over-training in increasing the risk of exercise-related injury.

2) List the symptoms of over-training.

3) Define acute and delayed-onset muscle soreness.

4) Discuss possible causes of muscle strains and ways in which they can be avoided.

5) Define tendonitis and discuss how it should be treated.

6) Discuss ligament sprains and how to avoid them.

7) Describe the most common injuries to the lower extremities.

8) Outline a general plan to reduce the incidence of exercise-related injuries.

9) Discuss the general guidelines for the treatment of injuries.

10) Define cryokinetics and discuss its use in the rehabilitation process.

LECTURE OUTLINE

Key Points	Subpoints	Examples
Risk of injury times body	1. 60% of running injuries are to the foot and knee	Reason: running stress is 2.5 weight
	2. Factors associated with running injuries	Improper training technique, shoes, alignment abnormalities
Common injuries	1. Back Pain	Causes: improper lifting, weak muscles, poor posture, bone disorders. Prevention: increase strength and flexibility of trunk flexors and extensors, reduce body fat.
	2. Acute muscle soreness	Cause: intense exercise. Prevention: Warm-up and cool-down, avoid excess intensity exercise.
	3. Delayed-onset muscle soreness	Cause: microscopic tears in muscle. Prevention: refrain from prolonged or intense exercise.
	4. Muscle strains	Cause: overstretched muscles. Prevention: Avoid loads that overstretch muscles.
	5. Tendonitis	Cause: Inflammation usually caused by overuse. Prevention: Avoid overuse.
	6. Ligament sprains	Cause: damage to ligaments. Prevention: Avoid activities that stress joints (tennis, soccer, running, etc.)
	7. Torn cartilage	Cause: high forces or unusual movements in joints. Prevention: Avoid activities that stress joints (tennis, soccer, running, etc.)
	8. Patella-Femoral Pain	Cause: overuse and misalignment of knee extensor muscles.

Key Points	Subpoints	Examples
		Prevention: Avoid activities that stress joints (tennis, soccer, running, etc.)
	9. Shin splints	Cause: inflammation between tibia and fibula caused by irritation from overuse. Prevention: run on soft surfaces, wear good shoes, slowly increase training intensity.
	10. Stress fractures	Cause: high stress or overuse causes fractures of bones (usually in foot). Prevention: avoid overuse, see physician for arch supports.
Reducing risk of injuries	1. Strengthen muscles	Maintain balance around joints
	2. Warm-up and cool-down	Remember stretching
	3. Use proper equipment	Shoes
	4. Do not overtrain!	Start low and progress slow
	5. Allow adequate recovery	
Management of injuries	1. Initial treatment	R - rest, I - ice, C - compression, E - elevation
	2. Rehabilitation	Cryokinetics

LAB ACTIVITIES

LABORATORY 11.1   (Page 267)
Students should complete the *Prevention of Injuries during Exercise* laboratory (Laboratory 11.1). The purpose of this exercise is find and eliminate ways in which your exercise program may cause injuries.

DISCUSSION ACTIVITIES
- Have students discuss injuries they have experienced and how they coped. What should they have done to manage the injuries?

• Discuss injuries most common to various sports and how they may be minimized.

SUGGESTED STUDENT ACTIVITIES
• Have an athletic trainer talk to the class about prevention and treatment of injuries.
• Have students visit a sports medicine clinic to observe professional treatment of injuries.

SUGGESTED READINGS

Jones, B.H., Harris, J.M., Vinh, T.N., and Rubin, C. Exercise-induced Stress Fractures and Stress Reactions of Bone: Epidemiology, Etiology, and Classification. In: Exercise and Sports Sciences Review. 17: 379-422, 1989.

Kibler, W.B., Chandler, J, and Stracener, E.S. Musculoskeletal Adaptations and Injuries Due to Over-training. In: Exercise and Sports Sciences Review. 20:99-126, 1992.

Neiman, David C. Fitness and Sports Medicine: An Introduction. Bull Publishing Co., Palo Alto, CA. 1990

EXAM QUESTIONS

MULTIPLE CHOICE

1. The impact of the foot on a running surface is approximately _____ times body weight.
   a. 2.5
   b. 5
   c. 7.5
   d. 10
   Answer: a, page 232, factual

2. Which of the following factors are associated with running injuries:
   a. shoes
   b. improper training techniques
   c. alignment abnormalities
   d. all of the above
   Answer: d, page 252, factual

3. Too much exercise and not enough recovery time is referred to as:
   a. supercompensation
   b. over-training syndrome
   c. fartlek training
   d. DOMS
   Answer: b, page 252, factual

4. To prevent the over-training syndrome, it is suggested that you increase your exercise intensity by no more than _____.
   a. 20% over a 2 week period
   b. 10% over a 2 week period
   b. 20% over a 4 week period
   d. 10% over a 4 week period
   Answer: b, page 252, factual

5. In aerobic dance, injuries occur at a rate of approximately:
   a. 1 / 50 hours of dancing
   b. 1 / 100 hours of dancing
   c. 1 / 150 hours of dancing
   d. 1/ 200 hours of dancing
   Answer: b, page 252, factual

6. Which of the following would be considered a primary cause of injury in aerobic dance?
   a. intensity of workout
   b. nonresilient surfaces
   c. duration of workout
   d. all of the above
   Answer: b, page 253, factual

7. Back pain is related to which of the following:
   a. disorders in the bones of the spine and back
   b. strength balance in hip flexors and extensors
   c. bed rest
   d. aerobic exercise
   Answer: a, page 253, factual

8. Which of the following plays a major role in prevention of back pain?
   a. exercise
   b. increasing body fat
   c. reducing hip flexibility
   d. all of the above
   Answer: a, page 254, factual

9. Pain developing immediately after exercise that has been too long or intense is referred to as:
   a. delay-onset muscle soreness
   b. acute muscle soreness
   c. over-training syndrome
   d. none of the above
   Answer: b, page 255, factual

10. Pain developing 24-48 hours after exercise is referred to as:
    a. delay-onset muscle soreness
    b. acute muscle soreness

c. over-training syndrome
d. none of the above
Answer: a, page 255, factual

11. Muscles which are overstretched or forced to shorten against a heavy weight are susceptible to:
    a. sprains
    b. tendonitis
    c. cartilage damage
    d. strains
    Answer: d, page 256, factual

12. The primary means of preventing ligament sprains is to:
    a. wear a joint brace
    b. consume large amounts of protein
    c. avoid intense exercise
    d. refrain from activities which place a strain on joints.
    Answer: d, page 257, factual

13. Patella-femoral pain syndrome is caused by:
    a. overuse
    b. overweight
    c. both of the above
    d. none of the above
    Answer: c, page 260, factual

14. Which of the following can help prevent shin splints?
    a. run on a soft surface
    b. wear well-padded shoes
    c. slowly advance exercise intensity
    d. all of the above
    Answer: d, page 261, factual

15. Which of the following refers to bones which crack due to the stress of excess load or duration?
    a. sprains
    b. strains
    c. stress fracture
    d. shin splints
    Answer: c, page 261, factual

16. Which of the following are considered ways to reduce your risk of injury during exercise?
    a. strengthen muscles
    b. increase intensity quickly to cause adaptation
    c. minimize recovery time
    d. do not increase flexibility of joints used in exercise
    Answer: b, page 255, factual

17. Which of the following is included in the R.I.C.E. treatment regimen?
    a. ice
    b. massage
    c. heat
    d. all of the above
    Answer: a, page 262, factual

18. The use of R.I.C.E. and exercise is called:
    a. message
    b. chondromalacia
    c. cryokinetics
    d. none of the above
    Answer: b, page 263, factual

TRUE / FALSE
19. The impact of the foot on the running surface is approximately 10 times body
    weight.
    a. True
    b. False
    Answer: b, page 252, factual

20. The primary factor associated with running injuries is improper training
    techniques.
    a. True
    b. False
    Answer: a, page 252, factual

21. Over-training syndrome results from too much exercise in relation to recovery time.
    a. True
    b. False
    Answer: a, page 252, factual

22. One of the primary causes of injuries in aerobic dance is improper shoes.
    a. True
    b. False
    Answer: a, page 252, factual

23. Back pain is due to many factors such as bone disorders and poor posture.
    a. True
    b. False
    Answer: a, page 253, factual

24. Strength balance of hip flexors and extensors is a primary means of preventing
    back pain.
    a. True
    b. False
    Answer: a, page 254, factual

25. Acute muscle soreness refers to pain occurring 24-48 hours after exercise.

a. True
b. False
Answer: b, page 255, factual

26. Prevention of acute muscle soreness could be accomplished by a slow progression of exercise training intensity.
a. True
b. False
Answer: a, page 255, factual

27. Prevention of delayed-onset muscle soreness can be accomplished by lowering training intensity and duration.
a. True
 b. False
Answer: a, page 255, factual

28. Strains are associated with stretched or damaged ligaments.
a. True
b. False
Answer: b, page 256, factual

29. Tendonitis refers to the soreness due to tears and damage to overused muscle.
a. True
b. False
Answer: b, page 257, factual

30. Sprains can be classified according to the degree of damage as a 1st, 2nd, or 3rd degree sprain.
a. True
 b. False
Answer: a, page 257, factual

31. Patella-femoral pain syndrome is also called chondromalacia.
a. True
b. False
Answer: a, page 260, factual

32. Shin splints occur from stress placed on the lower leg causing bones to split.
a. True
b. False
Answer: b, page 261, factual

33. Stress fractures result from the constant irritation to bones of the lower leg which results in inflammation of the muscles and tendons.
a. True
b. False
Answer: b, page 261, factual

34. The R.I.C.E. treatment utilizes heat and message to help rehabilitate injuries.

a. True
b. False
Answer: b, page 262, factual

35. Cryokinetics is another term for patellar-femoral pain syndrome.
    a. True
    b. False
    Answer: b, page 263, factual

DISCUSSION

36. Discuss the causes of injuries during running.
    Answer: page 252

37. Discuss the factors associated with over-training syndrome.
    Answer: page 252

38. Discuss the factors associated with chronic back pain and how may they be eliminated.
    Answer: page 253

39. Discuss the differences between sprains and strains.
    Answer: page 255

40. Discuss the differences in shin splints and stress fractures.
    Answer: page 261

41. Discuss ways of reducing the risk of injury during exercise.
    Answer: page 262

42. Discuss the R.I.C.E. principal and when it should be utilized.
    Answer: page 262

43. Define cryokinetics and discuss its use in injury rehabilitation.
    Answer: page 263

Chapter 12
Prevention of Cardiovascular Disease

CHAPTER SUMMARY

1. Heart disease is the number one cause of death in America. Almost one out of every two deaths in the U.S. is due to heart disease.

2. Cardiovascular disease refers to any disease that influences the heart and blood vessels. Common cardiovascular diseases include arteriosclerosis, coronary artery disease, stroke, and hypertension.

3. Coronary risk factors are factors that increase your risk for the development of coronary heart disease.

4. Coronary risk factors are classified as either *major* or *contributory risk* factors. Major risk factors are defined as factors that directly increase your risk of coronary heart disease. Contributory risk factors may increase your risk of coronary heart disease by promoting the development of a major risk factor.

5. Major risk factors for the development of coronary heart disease include: 1) smoking; 2) hypertension; 3) high blood cholesterol; 4) physical inactivity; 5) heredity; 6) gender; and 7) increasing age.

6. Contributory risk factors for the development of coronary heart disease include; 1) diabetes; 2) obesity; and 3) stress.

7. Your risk of developing coronary heart disease can be reduced by modification of the following risk factors: 1) smoking; 2) hypertension; 3) high blood pressure; 4) physical inactivity; 5) obesity; and 6) stress.

LEARNING OBJECTIVES

After reading this chapter, you should be able to:

1. Name the number one cause of death in the US.

2. Identify four common cardiovascular diseases.

3. Discuss the major and contributory risk factors associated with the development of coronary heart disease.

4. Identify which coronary heart disease risk factors can be modified by lifestyle alterations.

5. List the steps involved in reducing your risk of coronary heart disease.

6. Describe the link between dietary sodium and hypertension.

7. Identify total blood cholesterol levels associated with low, moderate, and high risk of developing coronary heart disease.

8. Discuss the relationship between diet and elevated blood cholesterol levels.

Lecture Outline

Key Points	Subpoints	Examples
Cardiovascular disease	1. Number one cause of death in U.S. in the U.S.	>69 million people have some form of heart disease
Cardiovascular diseases	Four common types: 1. Atheriosclerosis 2. Coronary heart disease 3. Stroke 4. Hypertension	

a. diabetes

b. stroke

c. hypertension

d. arteriosclerosis

answer: a, factual, page 272-276

3. Which of the following risk factors <u>is considered as a contributory</u> risk factors for heart disease?

a. cigarette smoking

b. hypertension

c. aging

d. diabetes

answer: ,d factual, page 280

4. Which of the following factors <u>is considered</u> to be a <u>major</u> risk factor for heart disease?

a. high blood cholesterol

b. obesity

c. diabetes

d. stress

answer: a , factual, page 280

5. Which of the following heart disease risk factors <u>cannot</u> be modified?

a. smoking

b. heredity

c. stress

d. hypertension

answer: b, factual, page 280

6. At present, heart disease is responsible for _____ deaths in the U.S.

a. one out of every two

b. one out of every three

c. one out of every four

d. one out of every five

answer: a, factual, page 271

7. Chest pain due to a reduction in blood flow to the heart is called
    a. a heart attack
    b. myocardial infarction
    c. angina pectoris
    d. none of above are correct
    answer: c, factual, page 273

8. If your experience heart attack symptoms for two minutes or more, you should
    a. lie down until the pain goes away
    b. run to the nearest hospital
    c. telephone the emergency medial service
    d. none of above are correct
    answer: c, factual, page 274

9.A stroke occurs due to
    a. blockage of a coronary artery
    b. blockage of blood flow to the brain
    c. blockage of aorta
    d. none of abve are correct
    answer: b, factual, page275

10. The cause of essential hypertension is unknown in approximately _____% of cases.
    a. 10%
    b. 30%
    c. 70%
    d. 90%
    answer: d, factual, page d

True/false
11. Arteriosclerosis is a single class of cardiovascular disease.
    a. true
    b. false
    answer: a, factual, page 272

12. Major risk factors for heart disease are defined as factors that increase your risk of
    heart disease by promoting the development of a secondary risk factor.

a. true

b. false

answer: b, factual, page 276

13. Coronary artery disease is the result of atherosclerotic plaque forming a blockage of one or more coronary arteries.

a. true

b. false

answer: a, factual, page 272

14. Myocardial infarction is another name for a "stroke"

a. true

b. false

answer: b, factual, page 273

15. A cardiovascular disease is any disease that affects the heart or blood vessels.

a. true

b. false

answer: a, factual, page

16. Uncomfortable pressure in the chest or dizziness are considered potential warning signals for a heart attack.

a. true

b. false

answer: a, factual, page 274

17. Clinically, high blood pressure is defined as a systolic blood pressure ≥ 140 mm Hg and a diastolic blood pressure ≥ 90 mm Hg.

a. true

b. false

answer: a, factual, page 275

18. One of the reasons that hypertension is a health risk is that chronic high blood pressure may damage the interior of blood vessels.

a. true

b. false

answer: a , factual, page 275

19. Smoking is not considered to be a major risk factor for the development of heart disease.
   a. true
   b. false
   answer: b, factual, page 276

20. Diabetes and heredity are both considered to be a "contributor" risk factor for the development of heart disease.
   a. true
   b. false
   answer: b, factual, page 277

21. Hypertension is considered to be both a disease and a risk factor for the development of heart disease.
   a. true
   b. false
   answer: a, factual, page 277

22. Another term for contributory risk factors is "secondary risk factors".
   a. true
   b. false
   answer: a, factual, page 277

23. When someone stops smoking, his or her risk of developing heart disease rapidly declines.
   a. true
   b. false
   answer: a, factual, page 277

24. Physcial inactivity is considered to be a major risk factor for the development of heart disease.
   a. true
   b. false
   nswer: a, factual, page 278

25. Blood cholesterol levels >240 mg/dl is considered to represent a low risk of developing coronary heart disease.
    a. true
    b. false
    answer: b, factual, page 278

26. Men have a greater risk of developing coronary heart disease than women.
    a. true
    b. false
    answer: a, factual, page 278

27. African Americans develop hypertension two-to-three times more often than whites.
    a. true
    b. false
    answer: a, factual, page 278

28. Smoking cigarettes, high blood cholesterol, and hypertension increases your risk of developing heart disease by almost 200%.
    a. true
    b. false
    answer: a, factual, page 278

29. Low-density lipoproteins are often called "good" cholesterol.
    a. true
    b. false
    answer: b, factual, page 279

30. High blood levels of high density lipoproteins reduces your risk of developing heart disease.
    a. true
    b. false
    answer: a, factual, page 279

31. Diabetes results in an increase in blood levels of glucose.

a. true

b. false

answer: a, factual, page 280

32. The distribution of fat on the body influences the risk of development of heart disease.

a. true

b. false

answer: a, factual, page 280

33. High sodium intake is not considered to be a factor in the development of high blood pressure.

a. true

b. false

answer: b, factual, page 281

34. Stress increases your risk of developing heart disease.

a. true

b. false

answer: a, factual, page 282

35. The four major risk factors that can be modified are smoking, hypertension, high blood pressure and diabetes.

a. true

b. false

answer: b, factual, page 282

36. Intake of saturated fats stimulate cholesterol synthesis in the liver and may therefore result in an increae blood cholesterol levels.

a. true

b. false

answer: a, factual, page 283

37. The two contributory CHD risk factors that can be modified are obesity and stress.

a. true

b. false

answer:a, factual, page 283

38. Saturated fats are found primarily in green and yellow vegetables.
    a. true
    b. false
    answer: b, factual, page 283

39. Heart disease is the leading cause of death in men between the ages of 35 and 44 years.
    a. true
    b. false
    answer:ab, factual, page 272

40. Hypertension is sometimes referred to as the "silent killer".
    a. true
    b. false
    answer: a, factual, page 276

Discussion

41. Identify the number one cause of death in the U.S. page 271

42. Define the following terms: pages 272-276

    cardiovascular disease

    coronary heart disease

    coronary artery disease

    hypertension

43. List the major and contributory risk factors for the development of coronary heart disease. pages 276-280

44. Discuss the difference between *major* and *contributory risk* factors for the development of coronary heart disease. pages 276-280

45. High density and low density lipoproteins have been labeled as being "good" and "bad" cholesterol, respectively. Explain? page 279

46. Which major coronary heart disease risk factors can be modified? page 280

132

47. Which contributory coronary heart disease risk factors can be modified?

    page 280

48. How does a high salt diet contribute to hypertension? page 281

49. What is the link between blood cholesterol and coronary heart disease?

    page 279

50. How does smoking increase your risk of developing cardiovascular disease?

    pages 276-277

51. How are arteriosclerosis and atherosclerosis related? page 272

52. Discuss the differences between a "mild" heart attack versus a "major" heart

    attack. pages 273-275

53. Define essential and secondary hypertension. page 275

54. Discuss the interaction between cigarettes, high blood cholesterol, and high

    blood pressure in increasing the risk for the development of coronary

    heart disease. pages 277-278

55. Why is increasing age a major risk factor for coronary heart disease?

    page 279

Chapter 13
Prevention of Cancer

CHAPTER SUMMARY

1. The group of diseases known as cancer are major killers and the incidence of these diseases are increasing. Currently, cancer is the number two cause of death in the U.S.

2. Cancer results from an abnormal growth of cells. This abnormal growth and division of cells forms a mass of mutated cells called a tumor. Tumors are classified as either benign (abnormal growth but not life-threatening) or malignant (cancerous cells that are life-threatening because they will eventually spread to other tissues and disrupt organ function).

3. Carcinogens are defined as cancer causing agents.

4. Skin cancer is the most common cancer. Other common sites of cancer include the mouth, lung, colon, stomach, colon, liver, bone prostate gland, and breast.

5. Normal cells become cancerous by damaging DNA which results in uncontrolled cell division.

6. Heredity, race, radiation, viruses, tobacco, alcohol, occupational carcinogens, ultraviolet light and a high fat diet are factors that increase your risk of developing cancer. Cancer risk can be lowered by reducing your exposure to radiation, tobacco, alcohol, ultraviolet light, and occupational carcinogens.

7. Approximately 80% of all cancers are related to lifestyle and environmental factors.

8. Diet is probably the most important factor in controlling your risk of cancer. Among the primary nutrients in foods that offer a protection from cancer

are vitamins A, E, and C. These nutrients reduce the risk of cancer by removing free radicals.

9. Exercise has been shown to reduce the risk of certain types of cancers.

LEARNING OBJECTIVES

After reading this chapter, you should be able to:

1. Discuss the incidence of cancer in the United States.

2. Define cancer.

3. Identify factors that influence you risk of developing cancer.

4. Discuss several types of occupational carcinogens.

5. List the most common types of cancer.

6. Outline ways to reduce your risk of skin cancer due to exposure to ultraviolet light.

7. Discuss the role of diet and exercise in reducing your cancer risk.

8. Explain how free radicals increase your risk of cancer.

Lecture Outline

Key Points	Subpoints	Examples
Cancer is the second leading cause of death in U.S.	1.Cancer will strike 3 out 4 families	30% of U.S. citizens will develop some type of cancer in their lifetime
Cancer is most common in older people		

Key Points	Subpoints	Examples
Warning signs of cancer	1. Change in size or color of wart	
	2. Sore that does not heal or heals slowly	
	3. Unusual bleeding from bowel, nipples, vagina, or presence of blood in urine	
	4. Thickening or lump in the breast or mouth	
	5. Indigestion that persists or loss of appetite	
	6. Obvious change in bowel or bladder habits	
	7. Nagging or persistent cough or hoarseness; or difficulty in swallowing	
Cancer is not a single disease but a class of 100 different diseases	1. Cancer is caused by an uncontrolled growth and spread of abnormal cells	Common types of cancer: Prostrate, breast, skin, stomach, etc.
Group of cancer cells is called a tumor	2. Tumors can be benign or malignant	
Causes of cancer	1. Cancer is caused by exposure to carcinogens-damaged DNA and cell division increases out of control	Common carcinogens include: radiation, chemicals, tobacco, etc.
Cancer risk factors	1. Heredity, race, radiation, viruses, tobacco, alcohol, occupational carcinogens, ultraviolet light, and diet influence your risk of cancer	Exposure to certain viruses, over-exposure to radiation increases your risk of cancer
Cancer prevention	1. Many cancers can be prevented by practicing a healthy life-style and avoiding chronic exposure to carcinogens	80% of all cancers are related to lifestyle and environmental factors

Key Points	Subpoints	Examples
Diet is probably the most important factor in cancer prevention	2. Vitamins A, E, and C may have a protective effect	These vitamins may offer protection against free radicals
Exercise reduces the risk of cancer	3. The mechanism linking exercise to a reduced risk of cancer is unknown	

LAB ACTIVITIES
LABORATORY 13-1, page 307

Laboratory 13-1 is a questionnaire that provides students an opportunity to increase their awareness of the risk of developing all forms of cancer. Answering yes to any of the questions on page 307 suggests that you should modifiy your lifestyle to reduce your cancer risk.

DISCUSSION ACTIVITIES

Organize a class discussion that centers on the importance of recognizing and reducing cancer risk factors. Focus the discussion on dietary issues (reducing fat intake, fiber in the diet,etc), limiting alcohol intake, and avoidance of cigarette smoke.

SUGGESTED STUDENT ACTIVITIES

Invite a health educator or a cancer research expert to discuss new research regarding the role of dietary antioxidants in the prevention of cancer.

SUPPLEMENTARY READINGS
American Cancer Society. 1993 Cancer Facts and Figures. Atlanta, GA, The American Cancer Society, 1993.

Bouchard, C., R.J. Shephard, T. Stephens, J.R. Sutton, and B.D. McPherson. Exercise, Fitness and Health: A Consensus of Current Knowledge. Human Kinetics, Champaign, IL, 1990.

Donatelle, R. and L. Davis. Access to Health: Brief Second Edition. Prentice Hall, Englewood Cliffs, NJ. 1993

Hales, D. An Invitation to Health. Benjamin/Cummings, Redwood City, CA, 1992.

Exam questions
Multiple choice

1. Cancer is a
> a. a single disease
>
> b. a collection of over 25 diseases
>
> c. a collection of over 100 diseases
>
> d. none of above
>
> answer c, factual, page 294

2. Agents that cause cancer are called
> a. drugs
>
> b. carcinogens
>
> c. transcription factors
>
> d. none of above
>
> answer b, factual, page 297

3. The most common type of cancer is
> a. stomach
>
> b. lung
>
> c. liver
>
> d. skin
>
> answer d, factual, page 294

4. A collection of cancer cells is called
> a. tumor
>
> b. cyst
>
> c. wart
>
> d. mole
>
> answer a, factual, page 294

5. Normal cells can become cancerous by
   a. damage to the mitochondria
   b. damage to DNA
   c. damage to the cell membrane
   d. none of above

   answer b, factual, pages 297-298

6. Approximately, ____% of all cancers are related to lifestyle and environmental factors.
   a. 20
   b. 40
   c. 60
   d. 80

   answer d, factual, page 300

7. Vitamins that may reduce the risk of cancer include
   a. A, E, and C
   b. K and D
   c. D and B_6
   d. none of above are correct

   answer a, factual, page 303

8. Which of the following is not a risk factor for cancer?
   a. radiation
   b. tobacco
   c. alcohol
   d. none of above are correct

   answer d, factual, page 298-303

9. Tumors that are considered to be life-threatening are called
   a. benign
   b. malignant
   c. cancerous
   d. none of above are correct

answer b, factual, page 294

10. Cancer is the _____ leading cause of death in the U.S.

    a. first

    b. second

    c. third

    d. fourth

    answer b, factual, page 293

11. The process of spreading cancer cells throughout the body is called

    a. hyperpolarization

    b. benign

    c. metastasis

    d. none of above are correct

    answer c, factual, page 294

12. Which of the following are not cancer risk factors?

    a) tobacco

    b) radiation

    c) heredity

    d) all of above are cancer risk factors

    answer d, factual, page 298

13. It is recommended that prior to sun exposure you apply a sunscreen with a
    sun protection factor of at least_____

    a) 10

    b) 15

    c) 25

    d) 30

    answer b, factual, page 301

14. _____ is probably the single most important factor in determining cancer risk.

 a) diet

 b) ultrviolet light

 c) alcohol

 d) radiation

 answer a, factual, page 301

True/False

15.Smoking is responsible for almost 75-85% of all lung cancer cases.

 a) true

 b) false

 answer a, factual, page 300

16. Research has shown that viruses are not linked to cancer.

 a) true

 b) false

 answer b, factual, page 298

17. Tobacco use is the single largest cause of cancer deaths.

 a) true

 b) false

 answer a, factual, page 298

18. Both the incidence of cancer and the cancer death rate are higher among whites than among blacks.

 a) true

 b) false

 answer b, factual, page 298

19. Diet is implicated in ~60% of all cancers in women and ~40% of the cancers in men.

a) true

b) false

answer a, factual, page 299

20. Heavy use of alcohol increases your risk of oral, liver, and breast cancer.

a) true

b) false

answer a, factual, page 299

21. Smokeless tobacco does not increase your risk of developing cancer.

a) true

b) false

answer b, factual, page 300

22. There has been a large increase in the amount of lung cancer in women since 1960.
a) true
b) false

answer a, factual, page 297

23. Cancer occurs when DNA is damaged and cell division increases out of control.
a) true
b) false

answer a, factual, page 297

24. The seven warning signs of cancer can be remembered as the word, "caution".
a) true
b) false

answer a, factual, page 295

25. The key to surviving testicular cancer is early detection.

a) true

b) false

answer a, factual, page 297

26. Almost all cancers occur in people over the age of 40 years.

    a. ture

    b. false

    answer a, factual, page 294

27. Almost 95% of all breast cancers are discovered by women themselves.

    a. true

    b. false

    answer a, factual, page 294

28. Testicular cancer is one of the most common cancers in young men.

    a) true

    b) false

    answer a, factual, page 294

29. Malignant melanoma is a dangerous type of liver cancer.

    a) true

    b) false

    answer b, factual, page 294

30. Cancer is the number two cause of death in the U.S.

    a. true

    b. false

    answer a, factual, page 293

31. Exercise has been shown to reduce the risk of certain types of cancers.

    a. true

    b. false

    answer a, factual, page 303

32. Cancer results from an abnormal growth of cells.

    a. true

b. false

answer a, factual, page 294

33. Among the primary nutrients in foods that may reduce your risk of cancer are vitamins K and B.
    a) true
    b) false

    answer b, factual, page 301

34. A potential sign of skin cancer is a sore that doesn't heal.

    a) true

    b) false

    answer a, factual, page 301

35. Free radicals can promote cancer by damaging DNA in cells.

    a) true

    b) false

    answer a, factual, page 302

36. Regular exercise has been shown to reduce your risk of cancer.

    a) true

    b) false

    answer a, factual, page 303

37. Vitamin E, C, and vitamin A are commonly called antioxidant vitamins.

    a) true

    b) false

    answer a, factual, page 303

Discussion

38. Define the following terms:
    cancer
    carcinogens
    tumor

page 294

39. What is the most common type of cancer? page 294

40. How do normal cells become cancerous? pages 297-298

41. List nine cancer risk factors. page 295

42. What is the "sun protection factor"? page 301

43. Exercise has been shown to reduce the risk of which types of   cancer?

page 303

44. What is an antioxidant? page 303

45. How do antioxidants reduce the risk of cancer? page 303

46. What types of cancer are linked to tobacco use? page 299

47. Name five occupational carcinogens. page 299

48. Discuss the signs of skin cancer. page 301

49. Outline the dietary guidelines to reduce your risk of cancer.

    page 304

50. Expalin how viruses can contribute to the development of cancer. page 298

Chapter 14
Stress Management and Modifying Unhealthy Behavior

CHAPTER SUMMARY

1. The five key health behaviors that promote a healthy life-style are: 1) health-related physical fitness; 2) good nutrition; 3) weight control; 4) stress management; and 5) modification of unhealthy behaviors.

2. Stress is defined as a physiological and mental response to something in our environment that makes us become uncomfortable. A factor that produces stress is called a stressor.

3. Two steps in stress management are to: reduce stress in your life; and to learn to cope with stress by improving your ability to relax.

4. Common relaxation techniques used to reduce stress include progressive relaxation, visualization, meditation, breathing exercises, rest and sleep, and exercise.

5. Behavior modification is the elimination of an undesirable behavior. The general model of behavior modification can be applied to achieve any desired health related behavior.

6. The five most common accidents are: automobile, fire, drowning, poisoning, falls.

7. Risk factors for accidents include unsafe attitudes, stress, drug use, and an unsafe environment.

LEARNING OBJECTIVES

After reading this chapter you should be able to do the following:

1. Discuss stress and stressors

2. Outline the steps involved in stress management.

3. List several common relaxation techniques used to manage stress.

4. Outline the general model for behavior modification.

5. Provide an example of how behavior modification can be used to modify
   unhealthy behavior.

6. Identify the most common types of accidents.
7. Outline steps to reduce your risk of accidents.

LECTURE OUTLINE

Key Points	Subpoints	Examples
Stress-impact on health	1. Stress is a major health problem in U.S.	10-15% of U.S. suffer from stress-related problems
Stress-defined	2. Stress is defined as a physiological and mental response to something in our environment that causes to become uncomfortable	Factor that produces stress is called a stressor
Stress impacts people in different ways	1. Personality type influences your response to stress (i.e. type A, B, or C)	Type A personalities have a heightened response to stress
Steps in stress management	1. First step is to identify factors that promote stress in your life and eliminate as many stress producing factors as possible	A classic example of stress that can be prevented is over-commitment (avoid over-commitment-practice good time management)

Key Points	Subpoints	Examples
Time Management	Guidelines to improve time management: 1. Establish goals 2. Use a daily planner 3. Evaluate your time management skills regularly 4. Learn to say no 5. Delegate responsibility 6. Eliminate distractions 7. Schedule time for you 8. Reward yourself when you complete a goal	
Coping with stress	Relaxation techniques: 1. Progressive relaxation 2. Breathing exercises 3. Rest and sleep 4. Exercise 5. Meditation 6. Visualization	
Modifying unhealthy behavior	General steps in behavior modification: 1. Identify problem 2. Desire change 3. Analyze history of problem 4. Establish shor- term goals 5. Establish long-term goals 6. Sign contract 7. Identify strategy for change 8. Use strategy and learn new coping skills to deal with problem	Examples of behavior modification include: 1. Smoking cessation 2. Controlling eating; weight control 3. Reducing risk of accidents

Key Points	Subpoints	Examples
Accidents	1. Number one killer of people under age of 35 years	Most common accidents: Automobile Falls Poisoning Drowning Fire
Reducing your risk of accidents	Take steps to reduce your risk of accidents in these key areas: 1. Reduce your risk of bicycle or motorcycle accidents 2. Reduce your risk of automobile accidents 3. Reduce your risk of injury due to fire 4. Take steps to reduce your risk of water-related accidents	

LAB ACTIVITIES

LABORATORY 14-1, page 327
LABORATORY 14-2, page 329

Laboratory 14-1 is a stress index questionnaire that is designed to increase student awareness of stress in their lives. Laboratory 14-2 contains a blank as well as a sample behavior modification contract. This lab presents the concept of how written contracts are useful in promoting behavioral modification.

DISCUSSION ACTIVITIES

This chapter provides several interesting topics for class discussion. Potential topics for class discussion include:

a) discuss the role of chronic stress in the development of both physical and mental disorders.

b) discuss the three primary personality types

c) discuss techniques for stress management

SUGGESTED STUDENT ACTIVITIES

Invite an expert on behavior modification and/or stress management to speak to the class on techniques to reduce stress via behavior modification.

SUPPLEMENTARY READINGS

Donatelle, R. and L. Davis. Brief Second Edition to Access to Health. Prentice Hall, Englewood Cliffs, 1993.

Howley, E. and B. D. Franks. Health Fitness: Instructors Handbook. Human Kinetics Publishers, Champaign, Illinois. 1992.

Margen, S. et al. (Eds.) The wellness encyclopedia. Houghton Mifflin Company, Boston, 1991.

EXAM QUESTIONS

Multiple choice

1. Which of the following is not considered to be a key health behavior?

   a. good nutrition

   b. weight control

   c. stress management

   d. none of above are correct

   answer: d , factual, page 311

2. A physiological and mental response to something in your environment that makes you uncomfortable is defined as

   a. stress

   b. stressor

   c. eustress

   d. hypostress

   answer: a , factual, page 312

3. A factor that produces stress is called

    a. eustress

    b. hypostress

    c. stressor

    d. none of above are correct

    answer: c , factual, page 312

4. A potential negative health effect of stress is

    a. lowered blood pressure

    b. increased mental alertness

    c. lowered disease resistance

    d. increased plasma volume

    answer: c , factual, page 312

5. Eustress refers to

    a. high stress levels leading to disease

    b. low stress levels leading to impaired performance

    c. stress levels that lead to improved performance

    d. none of above are correct

    answer: c , factual, page 313

6. People with type B personalities are generally

    a. impatient and aggressive

    b. hostile

    c. overweight

    d. easygoing

    answer: d , factual, page 314

7. The first step in behavior modification is to

    a. identify the problem

    b. desire change

    c. establish short-term goals

    d. none of above are correct

    answer: a , factual, page 320

8. In the U.S. _____ is/are the number one killer of people under the age of 35.

    a. heart disease

    b. cancer

    c. AIDS

    d. accidents

    answer: d , factual, page 321

True/False

10. Studies suggest that 10-15% of all U.S. adults may be functioning below optimal levels due to stress.

    a) true

    b) false

    answer: a , factual, page 311

11. Stress-related problems result in annual losses of billions of dollars to both businesses and government.

    a) true

    b) false

    answer: a , factual, page 311

12. The factor that produces stress is called eustress.

    a) true

    b) false

    answer: b , factual, page 312

13. Chronic stress can lower arterial blood pressure.

    a) true

    b) false

    answer: b , factual, page 312

14. From a medical perspective, stress can impact both physical and emotional stress.

    a) true

    b) false

    answer: a , factual, page 312

15. Eustress is defined as a level of stress that results in improved performance.

a) true

b) false

answer: a , factual, page 313

16. Type A personalities have a limited response to stress.

a) true

b) false

answer: a , factual, page 313

17. Type B personalities generally do not respond greatly to stress.

a) true

b) false

answer: a , factual, page 313

18. Type C personalities are generally highly competitive.

a) true

b) false

answer: a , factual, page 314

19. A classic example of stress that can be avoided is overcommitment.

a) true

b) false

answer: a , factual, page 314

20. Nutritional supplements have been shown to reduce stress.

a) true

b) false

answer: b , factual, page 315

21. Breathing exercises are a simple means of achieving relaxation.

a) true

b) false

answer: a , factual, page 315

22. Low to moderate intensity aerobic exercise has been shown to reduce stress.

a) true

b) false

answer: a , factual, page 316

23. Visualization is a technique that uses mental pictures to promote relaxation.
    a) true
    b) false
    answer: a , factual, page 319

24. The first step in behavior modification is to establish short-term goals.
    a) true
    b) false
    answer: b , factual, page 320

25. A potential cause of smoking is "social learning".
    a) true
    b) false
    answer: a , factual, page 321

26. Accidents account for 70% of all childhood deaths in the U.S.
    a) true
    b) false
    answer: a , factual, page 321

27. An important accident risk factor is an unsafe attitude.
    a) true
    b) false
    answer: a , factual, page 321

28. Stress can increase your risk of accidents.
    a) true
    b) false
    answer: a, factual, page 322

Discussion

29. Define the terms "stress" and "stressor". page 313

30. How do stress and eustress differ? page 313

31. Why is stress management important to health? page 312

32. List the steps in stress management. page 313-314

33. Identify some common stress management (relaxation) techniques. pages
    315-319

34. Define "behavior modification". page 319

35. What are the steps in behavior modification? pages 319-320

36. Outline a plan to use behavior modification to eliminate a specific unhealthy
    behavior. pages 320-321

37. Discuss the concept of eustress. page 313

38. Explain how exercise is useful in reducing stress. page 316

39. List the key guidelines for the development of a time management program.
    page 316

40. List the steps to reduce your risks of injury due to: automobile accidents;

falls, fires, falls, water accidents, and poisoning. page 321-323

155

Key Points	Subpoints	Examples
	1. Gonorrhea--caused from a bacterial infection; treated with antibiotics	~ 2 million new cases of gonorrhea occur each year in U.S.
	2. Venereal warts-caused by papilloma viruses; treated by surgery or topical medication to dry up the wart	Incidence is not well documented; however, veneral warts are common
	3. Herpes-caused by viral infections; no cure at present	Over one-half million new cases reported each year in U.S.
	4. Syphilis-caused by a bacterial infection; treated with antibiotics	~ 300,000 new cases reported in U.S. each year
Reducing your risk for sexually transmitted diseases	Guidelines for reducing your risk of STD's 1. Avoidance of contact with infected person-only absolute means of preventing STD's 2. Avoid causal sexual partners 3. Avoid using drugs or alcohol 4. Always practice safe sex 5. Never share hypodermic needles with anyone 6. Avoid oral sex or any activity where body fluids can penetrate through the skin	
Drug abuse	1. One of largest problems in U.S. today	Millions of Americans abuse alcohol and use illegal drugs

Key Points	Subpoints	Examples
Most commonly abused drugs in U.S. include alcohol, marijuana, and cocaine and cocaine	1. All three drugs have negative health consequences	Alcohol abuse may lead to liver damage Marijuana abuse may lead to lung diseases Cocaine abuse can lead to death due to cardiac dysfunction
Alcohol use students	1. Alcohol-most commonly used drug in U.S. 2. Alcohol abuse can lead to many health problems 3. Alcohol is a central nervous system depressant	85% of college use alcohol and 20-25% abuse
Marijuana use	1. Marijuana use became popular in U.S. in 1960's 2. Marijuana is classified as a stimulant	Most popular illegal drug on college campuses
Cocaine use	1. Cocaine use on the rise 2. Cocaine is a powerful stimulant	Estimated that 5 million Americans use the drug
Say "No" to drugs	1. Avoiding drug abuse requires discipline and control 2. Several steps can protect you from drug use: a) Increase your self-esteem b) Learn how to cope with stress	

c) Develop numerous interests

d) Practice assertiveness

LAB ACTIVITIES
Laboratory 15.1 page 343
This laboratory is designed to increase student awareness of their drinking habits.

DISCUSSION ACTIVITIES
Organize class discussions to emphasize the importance of "safe sex" in the prevention of sexually transmitted diseases. Also, conduct class discussions around the health and safety importance of avoiding drug use and alcohol abuse.

SUGGESTED STUDENT ACTIVITIES
Invite guest speakers to the class to discuss 1) the spread of AIDS in the U.S. and/or 2) the growth of drug and alcohol drug and alcohol abuse in the U.S.

SUPPLEMENTARY READINGS
Donatelle, R. and L. Davis. Brief Second Edition to Access to Health. Prentice Hall, Englewood Cliffs, 1993.

Margen, S. et al. (Eds.) The Wellness Encyclopedia. Houghton Mifflin Company, Boston, 1991.

Nevid, J. 201 Things You Should Know About AIDS. Allyn and Bacon, Boston, 1993.

Exam questions
Multiple choice
1. More than _____ different sexually transmitted diseases have been identified.

    a. 5

    b. 10

    c. 15

    d. 20

    answer d , factual, page 333

2. AIDS is a fatal disease that developes from a _____ infection.

    a. yeast

    b. bacteria

c. virus

d. none of above are correct

answer c, factual, page 333

3. Chlamydia is a sexually transmitted disease that is caused by a _____ infection.

    a. yeast

    b. bacteria

    c. virus

    d. none of above are correct

    answer b, factual, page 334

4. Gonorrhea is caused by a _____ infection that can be sexually transmitted.

    a. bacterial

    b. viral

    c. yeast

    d. fungus

    answer a, factual, page 335

5. Which of the following sexually transmitted diseases does not require medical
    treatment?

    a. chlamydia

    b. venereal warts

    c. syphilis

    d. none of above are correct

    answer d, factual, page 333-336

6. The most widely used and abused drug in the U.S. is/are

    a. alcohol

    b. amphetamines

    c. cocaine

    d. none of above are correct

    answer a, factual, page 337

7. Chronic use of alcohol can result in

    a. liver disease

    b. damage to the nervous system

c. increased risk of certain cancers

d. all of above are correct

answer d, factual, page 337

8. The most common recreational drug used by college students in America is/are

a. cocaine

b. amphetamine

c. alcohol

d. marijuana

answer d, factual, page 339

9. Cocaine is considered

a. a relatively safe drug

b. to be addictive

c. to be non-addictive

d. none of above are correct

answer b, factual, page 339

10. Long term use of marijuana

a. does not result in psychological dependence

b. can result in psychological dependence

c. presents no serious health risks

d. none of above are correct

answer b, factual, page 339

True/False

11. At present, there is no cure for AIDS.

a. true

b. false

answer a, factual, page 334

12. HIV can be transmitted by exchange of any body fluids.

a. true

b. false

answer a , factual, page 334

13. AIDS is caused by a viral infection.
    a. true
    b. false
    answer a, factual, page 333-334

14. Chlamydia is a sexually transmitted disease caused by a viral infection.
    a. true
    b. false
    answer b, factual, page 334

15. Pelvic inflamatory disease can occur in women due to untreated chlamydia.
    a. true
    b. false
    answer a, factual, page 334

16. Gonorrhea can be transmitted by vaginal, anal, or oral sex.
    a. true
    b. false
    answer a, factual, page 335

17. Over 80% of men infected with gonorrhea develop symptoms within 2-5 days.
    a. true
    b. false
    answer a, factual, page 335

18. Only 20% of women infected with gonorrhea develop symptoms.
    a. true
    b. false
    answer a, factual, page 335

19. Veneral warts are caused by a groups of viruses called human papilloma viruses.
    a. true
    b. false
    answer a, factual, page 335

20. About 90% of all untreated veneral warts result in cancer.

163

a. true

b. false

answer   b, factual, page 335

21. Herpes is a general term for a family of veneral diseases caused by viral infections.

    a. true

    b. false

    answer   a, factual, page 335

22. Herpes can be transmitted by oral sex only.

    a. true

    b. false

    answer b, factual, page 335

23. At present, there is no known cure for herpes.

    a. true

    b. false

    answer   a, factual, page 336

24. Most sexually transmitted diseases can be avoided by following "safe sex" guidelines.

    a. true

    b. false

    answer   a, factual, page 336

25. Syphillis is caused by a viral infection.

    a. true

    b. false

    answer   b, factual, page 336

26. Early symptoms of syphillis include a painless sore called a chancre.

    a. true

    b. false

    answer   a, factual, page 336

27. When untreated, syphillis can spread to other organs of the body.

a. true

b. false

answer   a, factual, page 336-337

28. Chemically dependency is another term for drug addiction.

    a. true

    b. false

    answer   a, factual, page 337

29. Chronic abuse of alcohol can result in liver damage.

    a. true

    b. false

    answer   a, factual, page 337

30. Alcohol is classified as a "depressant drug" because it results in depression of the central nervous system.

    a. true

    b. false

    answer   a, factual, page 337

31. Cocaine is the most widely used recreational drug in the U.S.

    a. true

    b. false

    answer b, factual, page 337

32. A common problem associated with alcohol abuse is undernutrition.

    a. true

    b. false

    answer   a, factual, page 338

33. Marijuana is classifed as a stimulant.

    a. true

    b. false

    answer   a, factual, page 339

34. Long-term use of marijuana presents no risk of health problems.

165

a. true

b. false

answer   b, factual, page 339

35. Regular smoking of marijuana may result in lung damage similar to that associated with smoking tobacco.

a. true

b. false

answer   a, factual, page 339

36. Use of cocaine results in depression of the central nervous system.

a. true

b. false

answer   b, factual, page 339

37. Regular use of cocaine can result in addiction.

a. true

b. false

answer   a, factual, page 339-340

38. Increasing your sel-esteem is one means of avoiding drug use.

a. true

b. false

answer   a, factual, page 340

Discussion

39. List and briefly define the seven most common sexually transmitted diseases. pages 333-335

40. Discuss the growth of AIDS in the U.S. Include in your discussion the relative increase in the number of AIDS patients over the past 10 years. page 334

41. Discuss the early symptoms of AIDS. page 334

42. Discuss the most common methods of transmission of AIDS. page 334

167

Chapter 16
Lifetime Fitness

CHAPTER SUMMARY

1. Exercise must be performed regularly throughout your life to achieve the benefits of physical fitness, wellness, and disease prevention.

2. Over 60% of the adults who start an exercise program quit within the first month. However, evidence exists that people who start an exercise program and continue to exercise for six months, have an excellent chance of maintaining a regular fitness routine for years.

3. The following factors are important in maintaining a lifetime commitment to physical activity: 1) goal setting; 2) activity selection; 3) regularity of exercise sessions; 4) monitoring your progress; 5) social support; 6) peers as role models; and 7) modifying your physical activity program as a result of aging.

4. Before choosing a health club, you should consider the following factors:

   1) Check the club's reputation with the Better Business Bureau before joining; 2) Investigate programs offered throughout your community before deciding on joining a particular club; 3) Before joining any facility, examine the membership contract carefully; 4) In general, avoid clubs that advertise "overnight" fitness or weight loss success; and 5) Arrange to make several trial visits to the facility before joining a health club. Several visits to the facility will provide you with answers to such questions as: a) are the locker room facilities well maintained and clean?; b) are the exercise machines in good working order?; c) are the club employees well trained and eager to answer your fitness-related questions?; and d) is the facility overcrowded during the hours that you plan to use the club?

5. There is no standard definition of a fitness expert. However, someone can generally

    be considered a fitness expert if they have earned an advanced degree (M.S. or

    Ph.D.) in exercise science, kinesiology, or exercise physiology.

6. Numerous exercise misconceptions exist. After studying this book you should be

    able to distinguish between fact and fiction. If you have doubts about the validity

    of a new fitness product or textbook, contact a local fitness expert for advice.

LEARNING OBJECTIVES

After studying this chapter you should be able to:

1. Identify several factors that will assist you in maintaining a regular exercise program.

2. List key considerations in choosing a fitness facility.

3. Discuss the term "fitness expert".

4. Discuss several common exercise misconceptions.

5. Identify factors to consider when purchasing exercise equipment.

6. List several precautions for the use of hot tubs, saunas, and steambaths.

LECTURE OUTLINE

Key Points	Subpoints	Examples
First 6 months of an exercise program are important	1. Studies have shown that people who begin an exercise program and continue to exercise regularly for 6 months have an excellent chance of maintaining a program for years to come.	60% of people who begin an exercise program quit in the first month
Maintaining a lifetime exercise program	Keys: 1. Strong personal commitment	

Key Points	Subpoints	Examples
	2. Establishing goals	Establish both short and long-term goals
	3. Selecting exercise activities that are fun	
	4. Properly planning exercise sessions	Establish exercise plans-follow your plan
	5. Monitoring progress	Maintaining a training log and periodic fitness testing are important
	6. Social support	Enjoying interaction with friends during a workout
	7. Peers as role models	Motivated peers who exercise regularly can be a positive influence
	8. Aging and changing physical activity needs	Need to modify exercise program as needed during lifetime-i.e. change exercise routine to meet changing exercise interest
Choosing a health club	Key points to consider:	
	1. Investigate the variety of clubs in your community	YMCA's, Wellness programs associated with college's and universities, etc.
	2. Check the reputation of the club or facility	See Better Business Bureau
	3. Visit the club several times prior to joining	Key questions include: Are locker rooms clean? Are exercise machines in good condition? Overcrowded?
	4. Check contract carefully before signing	
	5. Avoid clubs that advertise rapid weight loss	

Key Points	Subpoints	Examples
Diet and fitness products Consumer issues	1, Many common misconceptions exist about physical fitness	1. Yoga does not increase cardiorespiratory fitness and weight loss 2. Hand weights do not generally increase arm strength 3. Rubber suits or waist belts do not promote fat loss 4. Spot reduction of fat is not possible 5. Nutritional ergogenic aids do not promote physical fitness 6. Avoid exercise equipment that is advertised to promote rapid weight loss 7. Passive exercise machines do not improve physical fitness 8. Hot tubs, saunas, etc. do not promote fat loss 9. Carefully evaluate the credentials of authors of fitness articles or texts

LAB ACTIVITIES

There are no recommended laboratories associated with this chapter.

DISCUSSION ACTIVITIES

Discuss several factors that will assist individuals in maintaining a regular exercise program. Also discuss key considerations in choosing a fitness facility.

10. The first step in beginning a successful exercise program is the desire to be physically fit.
   a) true
   b) false
   answer a, factual, page 348

11. The second step in beginning a successful exercise program is to establish goals.
   a) true
   b) false
   answer a , factual, page 348

12. No single activity is excellent in promoting all aspects of physical fitness.
   a) true
   b) false
   answer a , factual, page 348

13. Choosing a regular time to exercise does not help in making exercise a habit.
   a) true
   b) false
   answer b , factual, page 348

14. Waterskiing is considered to be an excellent activity to improve cardiorespiratory endurance.
   a) true
   b) false
   answer b, factual, page 349

15. Monitoring your fitness progress is an unimportant factor in providing motivation to continue exercising.
   a) true
   b) false
   answer b , factual, page 349

16. Social support is a key factor in developing a successful exercise program.
   a) true
   b) false

174

answer a, factual, page 350

17. With aging it is important to modify your fitness program to meet your changing fitness interests.
    a) true
    b) false
    answer a, factual, page 350

18. Yoga has been proven to promote both physical fitness and weight loss.
    a) true
    b) false
    answer b , factual, page 352

19. Use of 1 pound hand weights during aerobic exercise (e.g. running) will promote large increases in muscular strength in most college age males.
    a) true
    b) false
    answer b , factual, page 352

20. The use of rubber waist belts will promote spot reduction of body fat.
    a) true
    b) false
    answer b , factual, page 352

21. There is a large amount of scientific evidence to support the notion that nutritional ergogenic aids will promote an improvement in physical fitness.
    a) true
    b) false
    answer b , factual, page 353

22. There are no "miracle" exercise machines that are capable of building huge muscles overnight.
    a) true
    b) false
    answer a , factual, page 353

175

23. Passive exercise machines have been proven to build muscle and to assist in rapid weight loss.
    a) true
    b) false
    answer b, factual, page 353

24. Hot tubs or saunas will not promote loss of body fat.
    a) true
    b) false
    answer a , factual, page 354

25. There are potential dangers associated with the use of hot tubs or saunas.
    a) true
    b) false
    answer a , factual, page 354

Discussion

26. Outline the key factors that play a role in maintaining a regular program of exercise.
    pages 347-350

27. List five points to consider when choosing a health club. pages 350-351

28. Give your definition of a fitness expert. page 352

29. Numerous exercise misconceptions exist. Discuss the misconceptions associated with Hatha Yoga, the use of hand weights, use of rubber weight belts to lose body fat, and nutritional ergogenic aids. pages 352-353

30. What factors should be considered when purchasing exercise equipment? page 353

31. List several precautions that should be considered when using hot tubs, saunas, or steambaths. page 354

32. Do passive exercise devices promote physical fitness and weight loss? Explain your answer. pages 353-354

33. What percentage of people who start an exercise program quit within the first month? page 347

34. Discuss the importance of activity selection in maintaining physical fitness. page 348

35. List five activities that are considered to be good or excellent modes to promote cardiorespiratory fitness. page 349

NOTES

NOTES

NOTES

NOTES

NOTES